Atlas of Difficult Gynecological Surgery

Anirudha Rohit Podder
Jyothi G Seshadri

Atlas of Difficult Gynecological Surgery

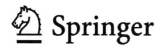

Anirudha Rohit Podder
Consultant Gynaec-Oncologist
Mahavir Cancer Sansthan
Patna
India

Jyothi G Seshadri
Department of Obstetrics
and Gynecology
Ramaiah Medical College
Bangalore
Karnataka
India

ISBN 978-981-13-8175-1   ISBN 978-981-13-8173-7   (eBook)
https://doi.org/10.1007/978-981-13-8173-7

This Springer imprint is published by the registered company Springer Nature Singapore Pte Ltd.
The registered company address is: 152 Beach Road, #21-01/04 Gateway East, Singapore
189721, Singapore

For
Guddu,
The only reason why I must keep trying,
My father, ***Sri. SK Podder,*** *and my wife,* ***Dr. Ruma Banerjee,***
For their unconditional love and for believing that I can do it
Reddy Bhai for making the photographs look better
And finally………….
Jyothi Madam, my coauthor and friend,
who encouraged me at every step

Preface

Why This Book?

The answer to this question, I suppose, cannot be given in one sentence. The purpose of writing this book is—.

I will try and answer this question a bit obliquely and hopefully eloquently. The health sector in our country is fast changing and so is the disease profile of most specialties. Gone are the days when a budding gynecologist could get an appointment order as a medical officer in a district hospital or as a faculty in a medical college soon after completing his or her residency or start his or her practice and hope to become a busy practitioner in about 3 years time. The concept of working under a senior consultant as an apprentice/clinical assistant does not exist in most parts of the country. Today vacancies are difficult to come by, and the logistics of starting one's own clinic in a decent locality with the present rental costs is not feasible for most beginners. In other words, the opportunities for higher training which have always been limited are getting even more difficult to get.

Also, the kind of cases we usually encounter in daily practice is changing. For many women, the first attempt at conception is probably their last. Many couples today are delaying having their first (and probably their only) child. An obstetrician-gynecologist has to remember that their patient may probably never conceive again, for obvious reasons like infertility (the present pregnancy itself being conceived through assisted reproduction), older age at conception, presence of leiomyoma, endometriosis, etc. This is one of the reasons why caesarean deliveries have increased. Rising caesarean section rate is not entirely wrong, but this has brought about many challenges. The management of second delivery, should there be one, and the management of gynecological conditions that may arise subsequently in women with a history of caesarean delivery have its own problems and challenges.

Rare conditions are no longer rare. It is just that their incidence is lower compared to the more common conditions. A practicing gynecologist is bound to encounter "rare conditions," a good couple of times during his/her career. Rude shocks on the operating table are common, and every operating gynecologist will experience them quite a few times in his/her career. Finding a malignant ovarian tumor or dense adhesions with complete distortion of the anatomy after opening the abdomen for what was thought to be a routine case of leiomyoma is no longer a rare case scenario.

So what should the operating gynecologist do in such cases? Is it possible to close the case and reschedule it later with adequate preparation and an experienced colleague to assist in all situations? This would certainly be a prudent thing to do if there is no complication like bleeding, but is it always possible? What about the gynecologist's credibility? Nobody would like to have too many "open and close surgery" in their list of surgeries performed. Or should one proceed with the surgery, even if one cannot find an experienced colleague to come over and assist? What if it is just not possible to comprehend what the pathology is, or where the surgical landmarks and the vital structures are located?

And another important development is that our society, maybe for justified reasons, looks at the medical fraternity with a certain degree of suspicion and disdain. People are not able to appreciate the fact that a great degree of skill is required to perform even minor procedures. It is not a mean achievement to perform surgical dissection close to vital organs like the ureter or the iliac vessels in a living being. And to acquire the skill and confidence to perform surgeries of this level, one has to put in many years of hard work. One has to go through the long learning curve, and one has to experience "complications"—for without this, one hasn't really seen or learnt anything.

For the reasons stated above, it is necessary for a doctor to be competent and efficient in all aspects—be it communication skills or surgical skills or decision-making, because litigation can happen even when the outcome is very good—much better than what is normally expected for the given case because it is suboptimal in the eyes of the patient. Very often, all what a doctor can do is say a few comforting words and provide a clean comfortable place so that the patients can breathe their last in peace and the family members are spared the agony of seeing their loved ones in pain.

Having said the above facts, let me come back to the basic question. Why this book? What is the need?

Well, we doctors in our daily grind forget that learning cannot be confined to our days in a medical college and attending training workshops. Learning is a continuous process. There was a time when a resident had to assist several cases as a second assistant before graduating to the position of the first assistant. The seniors would reward a resident who worked hard and managed cases well by allowing the resident to scrub in for a case. Teaching rounds were "real" teaching rounds, where the daily progress of each patient was discussed. The reasons for doing or not doing a particular investigation or procedure were discussed and debated. Unfortunately, critical evaluation of the self and of the system is on decline.

There is a lot of emphasis on "evidence-based medicine" today. But many a times, we need to follow what can be called the "best practices," especially in a low-resource setting where options are limited. Surgical "skill" and "technique" are not synonymous with evidence-based medicine. Skill and technique are things which have to be learnt, developed, and perfected over time. Constant evaluation of one's methods is a must for improvement, and this should not be confused with evidence-based medicine for or against a particular drug, or a particular kind of patient management. Can evidence-based medicine be quoted when the results are shockingly bad? Very often, the result speaks for itself.

For example, if there is traumatic PPH following vaginal delivery resulting in unacceptable morbidity for both the mother and the baby, can one justify the outcome by saying that there was no indication for LSCS? When we go through the medical literature, we will find that there are many schools of thought and rarely can there be one fixed protocol that everyone subscribes to. Every authority has had a unique experience, and there will always be a slight variation from one authority to another.

This book is essentially a compilation of some common sense facts; most of them are well-documented in all standard textbooks and are time-tested techniques, along with a few observations made by the author which should work for others as well. Beginners may not understand completely the description given in textbooks, even after they have read it a couple of times. It is only when one sees a senior gynecologist demonstrate a particular surgery live and explain the individual steps that one understands what the textbook description actually means. Demonstrating a surgery or a dissection technique is not the same as merely performing a surgery. It means patiently explaining the steps, allowing the surgical assistant to touch and feel the tissues and comprehend what is being done.

The techniques described in this book might appear very basic and in fact "child's play" to urologists, gastroenterological surgeons, and oncosurgeons. But considering that residents in obstetrics and gynecology get (and rightfully so!) a far greater exposure in obstetrics than gynecology, many gynecologists will find the techniques described in this book very useful and a bit of a revelation. The book has been written keeping in mind the Indian residency system—where every state, every region, and every university is different and there is a considerable variation in the residency pattern institution to institution.

And as a word of caution, nothing should be tried out like a recipe from a cookery book. It is necessary to have a good team while operating especially if it is expected to be a difficult case. This book is not a manual for all the surgical procedures described in obstetrics and gynecology till date. For this purpose, there are plenty of well-shot videos with excellent explanation available on the Internet and in private circulation which show how certain surgical procedures should be performed. This book, on the other hand, is strictly confined to the techniques which a gynecologist can follow when encountered with a sudden unexpected situation on the operating table. It is about the surgical dissection and some practical tips that are useful in optimizing the outcomes. For this reason, all the photographs in the book are of open surgery, since a beginner must first be able to perform a particular surgery and must be capable of identifying all vital structures in the operating field by the open method before attempting the same laparoscopically. This is not a book which tries to explain the etiology and pathogenesis, the medical management, the preoperative assessment, or the postoperative care of the various obstetric and gynecological conditions. It has been prepared with the intention to convince beginners the importance of good and careful dissection, the disasters that can happen due to ignorance and due to bad techniques, and, most importantly, that even the most complicated surgery can be successfully accomplished if one follows the "cardinal" rules. As stated earlier, this is not a self- help book, from which beginners can directly start operating on difficult cases. It is a book that hopes to make beginners understand *what, how much, how to*, and *in which manner* they should begin to improve their surgical skills and techniques.

Note: The word "obstetrician" has been used with respect to conditions pertaining to labor and delivery. The word "gynecologist" has been used with respect to other conditions described in the book. The doctors pursuing a career in "obstetrics and gynecology" are "obstetrician-gynecologists"—some of them end up practicing either of the two disciplines, some others a variable combination of both, and some specialize further in infertility, fetal medicine, etc.

Patna, India   Anirudha Rohit Podder
Bangalore, Karnataka, India   Jyothi G Seshadri

Contents

About the Authors

Anirudha Rohit Podder graduated from Bangalore Medical College, Bangalore, and completed his MS at Grant Medical College, Mumbai. He then trained as a gynec-oncologist at Gujarat Cancer and Research Institute (GCRI). Presently, he is working as a Consultant Gynaec-Oncologist at Mahavir Cancer Sansthan, Patna. Gynecological oncology and complicated gynecological surgeries are his areas of interest. He is a life member of the Karnataka State Chapter of Association of Gynaecologic Oncologists of India (KSC-AGOI) and has served as its joint secretary in the past. He has published articles in some of India's most prominent peer-reviewed journals.

Jyothi G Seshadri graduated from Bangalore Medical College, Bangalore, and completed her MD at Mysore Medical College, Mysore. She also holds a degree in Medical Law (PGDMLE) from the prestigious National Law School of India University. Presently, she is working as a professor at the Department of Obstetrics and Gynecology, Ramaiah Medical College, Bangalore. Passionate about preventive oncology, she pioneered the cervical cancer vaccination program at Ramaiah Medical College. She is a member of the BSOG and has served as its honorary secretary in the past. In addition, she has several publications in peer-reviewed journals to her credit.

Abbreviations

APTT	Activated partial thromboplastin time
CBC	Complete blood count
CPD	Cephalopelvic disproportion
D&C	Dilatation and curettage
DIC	Disseminated intravascular coagulation
DTA	Deep transverse arrest
DUB	Dysfunctional uterine bleeding
DVT	Deep vein thrombosis
ET	Endometrial thickness
FFP	Fresh frozen plasma
FHR	Fetal heart rate
GA	General anesthesia
GI	Gastrointestinal
ICU	Intensive care unit
IM	Intramuscular
IUD	Intrauterine contraceptive death
IV	Intravenous
IVF	In vitro fertilization
LSCS	Lower segment caesarean section
OT	Operating theatre
PCOD	Polycystic ovarian disease
PCV	Packed cell volume
PID	Pelvic inflammatory disease
PIH	Pregnancy-induced hypertension
PPH	Postpartum hemorrhage
PT	Prothrombin time
TOLAC	Trail of labor after caesarean
VBAC	Vaginal birth after caesarean
WBC	White blood cell

Part I

Introduction

Pressures of Being an Obstetrician-Gynecologist: *How Vulnerable Are We?*

1

The hallmark of obstetrics is that even the normal birthing process begins very often at the most "inopportune" time. And some of the most disastrous complications can happen suddenly with no warning, when one is just not prepared, and in some cases, in a perfectly normal patient. The specialty involves taking quick firm decisions. One must understand that other surgical specialties have the (relative) luxury of time for planning. One can keep the patient nil orally, wait for the availability of blood products to be confirmed, and can defer the surgical intervention at least till daybreak in most instances. But obstetricians have to do everything simultaneously; time is a luxury that they cannot afford. One cannot justify a bad outcome by saying "I waited for the vascular surgeon to arrive to begin the case because internal iliac artery ligation was required," "I waited for general surgeon/my senior colleague to arrive because the case was difficult," etc. Disastrous complications like fetal demise, uterine rupture, and progression from early DIC to irreversible shock can happen in a matter of minutes, even before blood investigation reports (CBC, PT, APTT) can arrive.

An obstetrician must explain the situation to relatives and take consent for the proposed procedure, convince the anesthetists about the urgency, arrange blood (well, where in the world can we expect 6 FFPs and 6 PCVs for the rare AB negative blood group to be available right away or for that matter arranged within 24 h), document the findings, give orders, call for extra helping hands, and inform ICU to keep a bed with ventilator ready-all in a matter of minutes. Though one may not practice high-risk cases, they are inevitable; every obstetrician-gynecologist will encounter them at some point of time. Sometimes seemingly normal patients deteriorate in a matter of minutes.

Though very often the intervention can be postponed for a few hours till daybreak or till a colleague arrives, this should not become a habit, a justification for obstetricians. Every case has to be individualized.

One must remember, postpartum hemorrhage requiring internal iliac artery ligation or hysterectomy, and a ruptured uterus with torrential internal bleeding are straightforward obstetric conditions. Expecting other surgeons to come at an unearthly hour to assist an obstetrician for what is an out-and-out an obstetric condition is impractical. Even medicolegally, it would be untenable for an obstetrician to defend his/her case by saying that a more experienced colleague was not around. A practicing obstetrician should be able to perform an emergency caesarean section even in the presence of conditions like thrombocytopenia, full-blown DIC, liver failure, heart failure, renal failure, etc. To work under pressure is a "given" for an obstetrician. One must call a fellow obstetrician for help and must

© Springer Nature Singapore Pte Ltd. 2020
A. R. Podder, J. G Seshadri, *Atlas of Difficult Gynecological Surgery*,
https://doi.org/10.1007/978-981-13-8173-7_1

simultaneously start moving-that should be the mantra.

Another dictum one should remember is that though normal delivery is the best for heart disease, DIC, severe pre-eclampsia, renal disease, or any condition where heavy bleeding is anticipated, it is better to do a neat and clean LSCS than a difficult vaginal delivery. For example, if the pelvis is borderline or if it is a case of previous LSCS [1, 2], it is better to do an LSCS when some blood products are available and experienced colleagues are around to help than performing it after a prolonged second stage when tissues are edematous and friable. It will be very difficult to suture the margins of a thinned out lower uterine segment, and the vaginal and perineal tears (in the case of a traumatic vaginal delivery), and the baby may also be born asphyxiated.

Another disadvantage an obstetrician-gynecologist must keep in mind is that when other surgeons encounter a sticky situation, they can very well manage it themselves, or by calling a senior colleague of the same specialty. So when an ophthalmologist encounters a problem while operating on the eye, he can manage it himself or by calling an ophthalmologist colleague. It is unlikely that he will ever need a neurosurgeon. Similarly, a ureteric injury when encountered by a urologist can be repaired by the urologist himself, a bowel injury encountered by a surgeon can be repaired by the surgeon himself.

But a gynecologist does not have that luxury. A rent in the posterior wall of the bladder, the bladder base involving the trigone, ureteric injuries, bowel injuries, and injuries to pelvic vessels, all require a surgeon trained in the concerned specialty. What a gynecologist must remember is that ureteric injuries in the pelvis are usually something that requires ureteric reimplantation since lower one third of ureter is the least vascular segment [3, 4]. It is a fact, something that has not changed over the years; gynecological procedures are the commonest cause of ureteric injuries [3, 4]. Similarly, injuries involving the large intestine might require colostomy since large intestine is poorly vascularized as compared to the small intestine. Transverse injuries to the mesentery, mesosigmoid, and mesocolon may require resection anastomosis since it means that the blood supply to the concerned segment of intestine has been cut off [5].

It is always better to plan a difficult case with an experienced colleague or another surgeon than call him midway for obvious reasons.

An obstetrician-gynecologist must always remember that unlike other surgeons, they are at a disadvantage because medicolegally they are not in a position to manage any injury involving the ureter, bowel, bladder, or the mesentery unless it is just a serosal injury of the bowel with no outpouching of the mucosa, a vertical tear in the mesentery with no purplish discoloration of the affected bowel segment of bowel, or a rent in the dome of bladder, not involving the posterior wall or trigone. One must call a more experienced colleague—a fellow obstetrician-gynecologist— to begin a difficult case, so that the injury can be avoided in the first place. One must prevent a situation where an injury has occurred due to carelessness or lack of expertise, and another surgeon has to be called midway. If it is known preoperatively that the disease involves the bowel or the ureter, like extensive endometriosis, and if bowel and ureteric surgery is required, then a surgeon or a urologist should be present right from the beginning. It is always preferable to call a fellow gynecologist with the experience and the expertise required for the particular case since a fellow gynecologist will be duty bound by ethics to be available in the event of any suboptimal outcome. Having a colleague of the same discipline is of immense support because the person will be involved with all aspects of patient care—patient counseling, fertility issues, etc. A fellow gynecologist can take charge if one is suddenly unable to manage the patient due to an unforeseen event like illness or a family emergency. But surgeons of other specialties will be concerned only with their territory. For example, a urologist will be concerned only with ureteric and bladder component of the surgery.

Should in situ findings turn out to be a complete surprise-something that was not suggested in preoperative assessment, then the gynecologist must immediately tell the relatives and quickly decide what the most prudent thing to do would be-to go ahead with the surgery by calling a more experienced colleague or close and reschedule the surgery with adequate preparation for a later date. But if a problem like bleeding or an injury has already occurred, it has to be managed appropriately then and there; there is no question of closing and rescheduling the surgery to a later date. But the incident must be critically evaluated at a later date.

References

1. Asfour V, Murphy MO, Attia R. Is vaginal delivery or caesarean section the safer mode of delivery in patients with adult congenital heart disease? Interact Cardiovasc Thorac Surg. 2013;17(1):144–50.
2. Kor-anantakul O, Lekhakula A. Overt disseminated intravascular coagulation in obstetric patients. J Med Assoc Thai. 2007;90(5):857–64.
3. Engelsgjerd JS, LaGrange CA. Ureteral injury. Treasure Island: StatPearls Publishing; 2018.
4. Burks FN, Santucci RA. Management of iatrogenic ureteral injury. Ther Adv Urol. 2014;6(3):115–24.
5. Mesdaghinia M, Abedzadeh-Kalaroudi M, Hedayati M, Moussavi-Bioki N. Iatrogenic gastrointestinal injuries during obstetrical and gynecological operation. Arch Trauma Res. 2013;2(2):81–4.

Which Incision to Take

2

The single biggest disaster that can possibly take place is directly opening the abdomen through a transverse incision, especially when the diagnosis is uncertain, or when the preoperative clinical assessment and imaging reports are only suggestive and not confirmative about the nature of the adnexal mass, or when there is a disparity between clinical examination findings and imaging findings. Even if another more experienced colleague is called midway during surgery, the disadvantage of having taken the wrong incision remains.

Per rectal examination in a woman with a pelvic/abdomino-pelvic mass is often forgotten mainly because its importance is underestimated. No doubt per vaginal examination yields more information. But the information that can be got by a per rectal examination is immense—the nodularity and fixity of the adnexal mass, whether rectal mucosa is involved or not, whether the pelvic mass is primarily of intestinal origin, should upper and/or lower GI endoscopy be done to confirm the exact nature of the mass, whether the ovarian tumor is malignant and is neoadjuvant chemotherapy preferable to staging laparotomy, whether the endometriosis involves the rectum— these are the points that can be fairly well determined by a per rectal examination. The information that can be got by the tactile sensation on our fingertips is something that no imaging modality can replace. This information is something that becomes more accurate with increasing years of experience.

Opening the abdomen through a transverse incision in an emergency situation can be justified in cases of ectopic pregnancy (laparoscopy would be ideal) and emergency caesarean section, no matter how complicated. Even when the presenting part is deeply engaged, when a classical caesarean section is planned or has to be done due to surprise finding of dense lower segment adhesions or leiomyoma, or multiple previous surgeries, when there is postpartum hemorrhage for which internal iliac artery ligation, or if caesarean hysterectomy has to be done, one can easily accomplish everything through a transverse incision by asking for general anesthesia and by converting the Pfannenstiel incision to a larger Maylard incision. If there is a surprise finding of an adnexal mass or an abscess during caesarean section, a transverse incision is still the rule since the additional procedure can be done through the same incision (if it is an emergency procedure like abscess drainage) or can be deferred to a later date with proper planning and preparation (like presence of a large leiomyoma or an ovarian tumor which requires staging).

Transverse incision for elective surgeries can be taken directly if one is very sure of the diagnosis—a straightforward elective caesarean section with nothing to suggest otherwise,

© Springer Nature Singapore Pte Ltd. 2020

A. R. Podder, J. G Seshadri, *Atlas of Difficult Gynecological Surgery*,

https://doi.org/10.1007/978-981-13-8173-7_2

hysterectomy for leiomyoma, adenomyosis, DUB, etc. But when the nature of adnexal mass is not known (the commonest disaster being finding an ovarian tumor in a patient opened up for a leiomyoma), or in cases of endometriosis—a condition which can be extensive despite the patient having no symptoms (indication for surgery could be for infertility), when there is a possibility of malignancy (sarcoma, ovarian tumor), when PID is suspected or is certain (there can be extensive adhesions involving the bowel), if the patient has had multiple previous surgeries, has received radiation or chemotherapy in past—directly opening the abdomen through a transverse incision is strongly discouraged. If one is lucky, then one might well be able to accomplish the surgery by requesting for general anesthesia (the surgery may have started with patient under spinal anesthesia) and by converting the incision to a much larger Maylard incision. If the condition requires staging or if upper regions of the abdomen are involved, then one might still be able to complete the case but one may have to confront a lot of complications a few days later. Bowel, bladder, and ureteric injuries can occur due to poor visualization and excessive retraction.

Small serosal injuries or a small cautery burn may heal by itself [1]. The patient may have to be kept nil orally for a longer period of time. Oral sips should be started only after complete recovery of bowel motility, that is, passage of flatus. The urinary catheter should be removed only after hematuria resolves completely, that is, urine microscopy should rule out microscopic hematuria. However, if larger injuries are missed, the patient may still be stable for the first day or two, but will deteriorate eventually. Bile or fecal matter may appear in the drain (if it has been placed) and the patient will develop peritonitis if a bowel injury has been missed. A urinary fistula will form if a ureteric or a bladder injury has been missed, and the patient will develop trickling of urine a week after the surgery [2, 3]. The appearance of blood in urine about 5 days after the surgery is a harbinger of this complication. Excessive retraction through a small incision will also affect would healing due to ischemic injury and pressure necrosis of the abdominal wall.

Bleeding vessels may be missed due to the same reason. The patient will have to be taken up for exploration in the very first postoperative day, if there is internal bleeding. Complications like rectus sheath hematoma are also known to occur because of excessive retraction of the abdominal wall [4]. In most cases hemostasis occurs due to the normal coagulation mechanism, the patient may still develop anemia in the postoperative period due to a missed bleeding vessel requiring transfusions, and this will result in escalation of treatment costs.

So when one encounters such a situation-abdomen opened through a transverse incision when a vertical incision would have been appropriate, the choice is between taking a vertical incision, which results in patient having an inverted T incision, or closing and deferring the case to a later date. The choice depends on the condition which has been discovered on table and whether the condition is an emergency. For example, for multiple pelvic abscesses which cannot be deferred to a later date, one has to proceed by taking a vertical incision and thoroughly drain the entire peritoneal cavity.

So what should be the correct incision? In the age of laparoscopy, we must use laparoscopy more often and as a diagnostic tool as well. Insert a laparoscope—it will provide an excellent panoramic view, and then decide how to go ahead—proceed laparoscopically, or take a transverse incision or a vertical incision.

One must remember that surgery is the ultimate diagnostic tool. Many conditions require exploration, which means we are opening to explore, to find out, and if possible to treat the condition that exists in the patient. One has to choose laparoscopy over laparotomy wherever possible, and one should never be embarrassed when a laparoscopic surgery gets converted into a laparotomy, especially if the exact nature and extent of the disease gets confirmed only after having inserted a laparoscope. Even in cases of large lesions, in patients with history of multiple previous surgeries, one can (and should) successfully insert a laparoscope through the open method and then insert the side ports under vision. Initial inspection by laparoscopy can be done even in cases where the patient has had one or more previous suboptimal surgeries.

So far the author has been able to successfully operate on all patients referred with a diagnosis of being inoperable. This is solely because a vertical incision was taken, while the primary surgeon attempted the same through a transverse incision. Both, midline vertical and paramedian incision are similar when it comes to exposure and ease of closure. However, midline vertical incision is cosmetically superior, if the incision needs to be extended above the umbilicus. One must skirt around the umbilicus if the incision needs to be extended. This is because umbilicus is a region rich in skin commensals, and infection of the wound around this region is very painful and disfiguring.

Paramedian incision involves cutting of the nerves, and this can lead to a slightly higher incidence of incisional hernia as compared to midline vertical incision. Midline vertical incision by virtue of being in the midline receives lesser blood supply and can heal poorly as compared to transverse and paramedian incisions [5].

References

1. Tsai MC, Candy G, Costello MA, Grieve AD, Brand M. Do iatrogenic serosal injuries result in small bowel perforation in a rabbit model? S Afr J Surg. 2017;55(2):18–22.
2. Lee JS, Choe JH, Lee HS, Seo JT. Urologic complications following obstetric and gynecologic surgery. Korean J Urol. 2012;53(11):795–9.
3. Tarney CM. Bladder injury during cesarean delivery. Curr Womens Health Rev. 2013;9(2):70–6.
4. Kapan S, et al. Rectus sheath hematoma: three case reports. J Med Case Rep. 2008;2:22.
5. Burger JWA, van 't Riet M, Jeeke J. Abdominal incisions: techniques and postoperative complications. Scand J Surg. 2002;91:315–21.

Anatomy: *How to Locate Vital Structures in Pelvis*

3

Residents are often told to read up on the surgery—indications, contraindications, steps involved, complications, etc., before they come to the operation theater to witness or to assist in a case. Many seniors proudly declare that they read all about the surgery before they come to the operation theatre even to this day.

But for beginners, it is only after they see the dissection happening live, only after they get to palpate the structures in a live surgery, are they in a position to understand what the textbook description actually means. To be the first assistant to a senior surgeon who patiently describes each step and allows a beginner touch and feel every structure is a unique learning experience that cannot be compensated by reading books or watching videos. It is possible to conceptualize and comprehend only when one is the first assistant and has seen a senior perform the surgical dissection live.

The first challenge in a badly distorted case is how to enter the pelvis, because the bowels are densely adherent to each other, to the anterior abdominal wall, and to the pelvic structures. Bowels can get injured while opening the peritoneum itself because the bowel loops could be adherent to the overlying peritoneum right under the incision site. This can be avoided by opening the peritoneum bluntly using fingers or preferably by holding a fold of peritoneum with two artery forceps about a centimeter apart. One

can then feel with thumb and index finger if there is any other structure felt below and open the peritoneum by making a small nick and then extending the peritoneal opening in the direction where there are no adherent underlying structure. In laparoscopy, one can insert the camera port by the open method and then insert the side ports under direct vision. Even in a badly distorted case, it is fairly easy to distinguish the small intestine from the large intestine. The presence of three white bands, teniae coli, that run along the length of the large bowel helps to distinguish the large intestine from the small intestine. The caliber of the bowel should not be the criteria. Even in gynecological surgeries, it is possible to come across a hugely dilated small intestine due to adhesions. The segment above the partial obstruction is dilated, whereas the intraperitoneal parts of the large intestine (caecum, transverse colon, sigmoid, and rectum), which lie distal to the point of subacute obstruction, can be collapsed and be of a smaller caliber than the proximal part of small intestine. The distinguishing feature is the presence of teniae coli. The large intestine can be collapsed and may be of the same caliber of the small intestine in patients who have been given a good preoperative bowel preparation. Therefore, the presence of teniae coli must be looked for. In some cases of PID, there can be a large hydrosalpinx—the fallopian tube can be hugely distended and can look like a segment of

© Springer Nature Singapore Pte Ltd. 2020
A. R. Podder, J. G Seshadri, *Atlas of Difficult Gynecological Surgery*,
https://doi.org/10.1007/978-981-13-8173-7_3

the small intestine. One has to be careful while dissecting and separating the structures; only after the dissection is complete, the fallopian tube can be identified by locating the fimbrial end. Sometimes the fimbria is not made out due to adhesions or pus. In such situations, the fallopian tube can be confirmed by noting that the entire lengths of the small and large intestines are separate from the fallopian tube (There may not be a uterus if the patient has undergone hysterectomy previously. So if the fimbrial end is necrotic, then there may not be a uterus at the cornual end).

And while separating the bowel adhesions, one has to be careful to dissect along the antimesenteric border, lest the mesentery, mesosigmoid, and mesocolon are trimmed away from the bowel segment. It is advisable to call another gynecologist with greater expertise in adhesiolysis, irrespective of his or her age for assistance. Remember calling another surgeon of a different specialty midway, when the dissection has begun and has its own problems. If the condition is entirely gynecological, it conveys a lack of skill in the gynecologist to other specialists. To patient's relatives, it will appear that the gynecologist has committed a blunder. *Has some problem or an injury occurred? Why is another surgeon being called now?* But calling a fellow gynecologist by and large will not create such an impression. It would only suggest that more assistance is required.

Not that one must not seek the help of other surgeons but first call a fellow gynecologist if possible. A fellow gynecologist with experience and expertise will know the gynecological indication for which the surgery is being done, for example, why is the adhesiolysis being done, does the patient wish to preserve her fertility, etc. A fellow gynecologist by virtue of being in the same specialty will be able to help the primary gynecologist manage the postoperative problems including handling patient's concerns. A surgeon of a different specialty will only be concerned with that limited territory alone. For example, if a urologist has been called to repair an injured

ureter, the urologist will follow-up with the repair procedure only. But had there been an experienced fellow gynecologist right from the beginning of the surgery, then the ureteric injury might possibly have been avoided. And the fellow gynecologist colleague will be duty bound to help the primary consultant with everything—postoperative problems, explaining the condition to patient and relatives, possible loss of fertility potential, etc. How can one expect a surgeon of another specialty to help in this regard? Why would any surgeon other than a fellow gynecologist be interested in issues like (loss of) fertility, future child bearing, etc.?

But as a note of caution, do not hesitate to call the right person, a fellow gynecologist or a urologist, or a general surgeon, but do not call a surgeon of a different specialty just because one fears competition, or because one does not want fellow gynecologists to know about one's cases.

When the anatomy is distorted or when tissues are friable or when there are dense adhesions, one must do sharp dissection and not blunt dissection. This is to be followed very strictly especially when one is close to vital structures. The logic being that a neat and clean cut is easier to repair. Never try to shell out what could be a segment of bowel. Never try to strip two layers of bowel stuck to one another or to the anterior abdominal wall. Or for that matter, never try to peel off a segment of bowel stuck to the uterus or ovary. The small intestine if torn can be repaired by closing in two layers or by resection of the damaged segment followed by anastomosis of the two cut ends [1]. The large intestine does not share the same privilege. Unless it is a very small rent, the general rule is colostomy, and this will not be an easy situation to handle. What if the patient is young mother, the only bread earner of the family, a young student preparing for an important examination, a deeply religious person who needs to go to a place of worship, a cook who has to enter the kitchen—How can a person with a colostomy perform these roles?

And remember, colostomy will need to be closed at a later date, which means another procedure under anesthesia. Closure of an intestinal rent without showing it to a surgeon is strongly discouraged (preferably call a surgeon to do the repair) ; it might result in leaks which will become evident on finding bile and/or fecal stained drain fluid postoperatively.

Another rule to be kept in mind is that one must not use cautery excessively and indiscriminately when close to vital structures. Check if the metal instrument is touching or is in contact with any other structure, or is it in contact with another mental instrument like the retractor before buzzing it. The thermal damage due to cautery extends well beyond the visibly charred area. Things may look fine at the time of closure, but the damaged tissues will slough away and a ureterovaginal fistula (evident by continuous trickle of urine in the vagina) or a bowel perforation with fecal/biliary peritonitis will occur about 5 days after surgery. Not just the viscera, even skin burns are known to occur leading to poor wound healing, due to carelessness while using cautery [2, 3]. If the forceps touches the metal retractor, there can be an extensive charring—remember the business end of the retractor can be broad, and the amount of avoidable damage can be extensive.

Do not apply clamps blindly and take deep stitches to secure bleeders without checking what is held in the pedicle. This is a common cause of ureteric injuries [4, 5]. Apply pressure with a mop. Hold the structures with atraumatic instruments—Babcock or an artery forceps. Then trace the ureter and make sure it is away from the bleeding point. And then apply cautery catching the bleeder points only, or take stitches or apply a free tie once it is certain that no vital structure is included in the pedicle. A less commonly encountered postoperative complication is a vesicovaginal fistula or a ureterovaginal fistula becoming obvious after the fifth postoperative day. The patient complains of watery leak or a continuous trickle of urine from the vagina. This is because a part of bladder, or the ureter, was damaged by cautery, or was included in sutures

during surgery. This most commonly happens when the bladder is not well separated during hysterectomy, and as a result has suffered thermal damage due to cautery being applied close to it's tissue, or because a part of it has been included in the sutures, or both. The damaged tissue sloughs away over the next few days, resulting in the formation of a fistulous track, usually a week after the surgery.

Therefore, identifying and repairing the damage during primary surgery is undoubtedly a better situation to be in than encountering a shock a week later (while all along one was feeling very happy for having accomplished a challenging case successfully). But better still would be to avoid damage to a vital structure in the first place by correctly identifying the structure before applying cautery or taking a stitch.

How to confirm the presence of a small bowel perforation? A fairly large rent is obvious. A generous amount of warm saline must be poured into the peritoneal cavity. Let the bowel loops submerge in the pool of saline. If one sees gas bubbles coming out, there has to be a rent in a gas-filled organ. Gas being lighter than water will come out and can be seen as bubbles in a pool of saline. Just like how puncture in a tire tube was located before the age of tubeless tires! This technique is also used by surgeons after performing resection anastomosis of the bowel. If air bubbles are seen coming out of the site of bowel anastomosis after it is submerged in a saline-filled kidney tray or pelvis, then it means that the anastomosis is not water tight.

In case of suspected rectal or sigmoid injury, fill the pelvis with saline and ask an assistant to blow a jet of air using an asepto syringe through the anus from below. If air bubbles are seen in the pelvis, it means there must be a rent in the rectum or the sigmoid.

Once the bowel loops have been separated from one another and the access to the pelvis gained, the intended gynecological procedure can be performed. During residency, gynecologists are taught very well the steps one should follow to avoid ureteric injuries. Most residents are very well aware of these by the end of their residency.

They are

- Do not go too laterally; apply clamps as close to the specimen as possible.

The most common sites where the ureter is injured are during the clamping of the infundibulopelvic ligament, the uterine artery, the uterosacral ligament, and the vaginal vault. Hence, one must stay close to the specimen, and all the subsequent clamps must be applied medial to the preceding clamps.

- Skeletonize the uterine arteries by incising both the utero-vaginal fold anteriorly and the posterior peritoneum. So when one applies the uterine clamp, one is sure that only the uterine vessels have been held and no other retroperitoneal structure.
- Separate the bladder and push it down. Ask the assistant to give moderate upward traction to the specimen; by doing so, the bladder and the ureters fall back and are less likely to be included in the clamps or sutures.

Well, it is a bit embarrassing for gynecologists that gynecological surgery is the most common cause of ureteric injury, and this has not changed over the years. So how does one locate the ureter? Unlike the small and large intestine, ureters are not intraperitoneal in any part of their course? Even in a case with no anatomic distortions, they can be exposed only by opening the retroperitoneum. If there are no adhesions or if there is no collection in the pouch of Douglas, they can be seen transperitoneally.

It is quite easy to locate and identify the ureters. One has to divide the round ligament, which has been described by many standard textbooks as the most consistent landmark in a female pelvis. Following this, one has to separate the two folds of the broad ligament extending laterally. Blunt dissection would be preferable at this stage, but not when the tissues are densely adherent to each other. One of the cardinal rules, never force open a space should be kept in mind.

The gloved fingers can be inserted, and the loose areolar tissues are gently separated. Once the external iliac artery is located, go upwards, and the ureter can be seen crossing the bifurcation of the common iliac artery. The ureter then runs medially along the fold of the broad ligament and passes below the uterine artery—water under the bridge; it then takes a sharp medial turn at the level of the ischial spine to enter the trigone of bladder.

The arteries are seen pulsating, whereas the ureter shows peristalsis if stimulated with a blunt atraumatic forceps. The question of confusing the ureters with a vein does not arise. The veins are blue, and the external iliac vein runs under the external iliac artery. Do not touch the vein with any pointed instrument. They being thin walled can tear, and a vascular surgeon will have to be called urgently. The bleeding, dark red in color, will soon fill the entire pelvis. Just put a mop and apply pressure, and call the vascular surgeon.

If the ureter is seen adherent to the mass/fibroid, then use sharp dissection. Ask for a tape and take the ureter on this and lateralize it. Remember; do not apply cautery on the ureter. Hold the bleeder with a fine tip forceps and lift it away from the ureteric surface before buzzing it. The tip of the forceps should be away from the ureteric serosa, while cauterization.

One instrument that gynecologists must use more often is the right-angled forceps, also called mixter. This instrument cannot be replaced by any other, or done away with. For many steps, like taking the ureter on the tape, passing the stout silk under the internal iliac artery for internal iliac artery ligation, mobilizing the ureter out of the tunnel of Wertheim, and sometimes even for adhesiolysis, right-angled forceps is a must.

One can also take the external iliac artery on tape (if the adnexal mass lies close to it), but never do that with a vein. There is an instrument called a vein hook to gently lift the vein and to expose its under surface. Remember there could be a tributary of the vein in the under surface which could get torn and lead to a very difficult situation.

Always feel the ureter with your thumb and index finger, sometimes the ureter can be better felt than seen. Some seniors describe the ureter as a cord that slips between fingers. Once this feeling is registered in mind, one will never forget the tactile feel of the ureters.

If ureteric or bladder injury is suspected, checking the color of urine for the presence of blood is not always reliable since blood-stained urine can happen even when there is extensive handling and due to rough retraction. Deaver's retractor is the preferred retractor for most gynecologists for pelvic surgery. Doyen's retractor on the other hand is suitable for caesarean sections. If rough handling is the cause of hematuria, then delayed removal of Foley catheter would be advocated since some amount of denervation might have occurred (e.g., if the ureters have been taken on a tape and have been lateralized). Bladder atonia/hyponia may result postoperatively, and the patient may not feel bladder fullness and may have difficulty in voiding. The author once had an unusual experience. In one case, there was blood in the urine bag, but no ureteric or bladder injury had occurred. This was during a case of radical hysterectomy. When urologists were called, they confirmed the absence of any injury. However, clots had formed in the bladder due to rough retraction by the novice second assistant. The clots were flushed out, and continuous irrigation of bladder was performed by placing a three-way Foley catheter.

To confirm any ureteric injury, one has to trace the ureters on both sides and look if any sutures or cautery burn marks are in the vicinity of the ureters. Gently stimulate the ureters with a blunt instrument and check for peristalsis. As mentioned before, the color of urine can be blood stained even without crushing, ligation, and transection injuries. A complete ligation of the ureter with a deep stitch is something that happens only when one holds a very thick chunk of tissue in a pedicle and takes a deep stitch without checking what is in the chunk of tissue which has been held. This is a very gross mistake, since one of the cardinal rules is never take a deep stitch in the pelvis without knowing what could

be inside the pedicle; one never knows what one could be ligating. Theoretically, this might not result in blood-stained urine because the entire lumen has been closed by a tight stitch, and the ureteric wall has not been pierced. But the urine output postoperatively will be very low, and the patient will have severe flank pain on the affected side.

Just as mere presence of blood-stained urine does not mean ureteric or bladder injury, the mere finding of low urine output also does not mean ureteric injury. Low urine output might be because of anemia and dehydration. Fluid replacement is usually underestimated. The total output from all the drains should be taken into account. If the output is at least one third the input, then it is reassuring, provided that the total urine output is at least 30 mL/h, or the 24 h urine output is more than 500 mL [6]. Also if the urine is concentrated, it means that kidneys are able to concentrate urine, it is unlikely ureters are injured in the absence of other findings. But remember, sudden appearance of hematuria a week after surgery followed by dribbling means a fistula, even if the patient had no specific symptoms immediately after surgery.

Locating the bladder is not difficult. Just try and locate the bulb of the Foley catheter. One can inflate the bulb with greater amount of distilled water, so that a hugely distended bulb can serve as a visible landmark throughout the surgery. If the Foley bulb is visible, then it is obvious that there is a rent in the bladder. But whenever a bladder injury is suspected, the time-honored technique of confirming the rent is to do retrograde filling with saline stained with methylene blue. If bluish saline is seen pouring into the pelvis, then there is no doubt that the bladder is injured [4, 5].

Call a urologist if posterior wall, trigone, or ureters are damaged. Only the dome of the bladder can safely be closed by the gynecologist himself/herself.

Now, should a gynecologist ask for stenting of the ureters prior to surgery in all difficult cases [4, 5]? Well, gynecologist must know how to locate and trace the ureters. The number of cases where the operating gynecologist will get rude shock on the operating table will be far more than cases where a prophylactic preoperative stenting has been performed for a broad ligament or a cervical leiomyoma. In many patients, preoperative imaging shows nothing to suggest a badly distorted anatomy. Is it advisable or feasible to prophylactically stent the ureters preoperatively in all cases? The answer clearly is no. The operating gynecologist must be able to locate and trace the ureter from the point of entry into the pelvis, that is, from the point where the ureter crosses the bifurcation of common iliac artery to the trigone of bladder.

Now, how do we locate the ureter in case of laparoscopy where we do not have the luxury of feeling it with our fingers? What beginners are taught is apply the grasper/harmonic as close as possible to the ovaries while cutting the infundibulopelvic ligaments. In case of large ovarian masses, this precaution alone might not be enough. Follow the same techniques, and divide the round ligament. Use a hook and split open the folds of the broad ligament, and enter the retroperitoneal space. Use a hook and separate the loose areolar tissues. Hook the tissue and lift it, making sure there is nothing under it. Once the ureters are located, safely catch the infundibulopelvic ligament. And if the case is difficult and one cannot call a more experienced colleague, never hesitate to convert it into a laparotomy. Never apply cautery blindly. In case of laparoscopy, remember the role of an assistant is much more than in laparotomy. One needs far more able assistants for laparoscopic surgeries than when compared to laparotomy. One cannot compromise by having a shaky hand holding the camera. The placement of ports should be correct. Instruments should never cross each other and create what is often described as "sword fight in the abdomen."

Now lastly, what to do when there is no round ligament? How do we locate the ureter in such situations where there is no visible trace of the round ligaments? This can be due to adhesions following previous surgery.

In such situations, hold a fold of posterior peritoneum in the lateral side of pelvis and feel with fingers if there is any tubular structure underneath. Make a small nick on the posterior peritoneum and open the retroperitoneal space. Gently extend the incision on the posterior peritoneum, making sure there is no structure underneath. Try to locate the bifurcation of the common iliac artery with ureter crossing it.

Lastly another time-honored dictum is in pelvic surgery, do not forcibly open a space and do not create a space, the bottom of which cannot be seen. Should torrential bleeding occur, it will be very difficult to control it. It may not be possible to open a space due to many reasons—previous surgery, radiation, presence of malignancy with parametrial extension (think whether has anything been missed out in the preoperative evaluation), induration due to pelvic infection, or maybe one is simply not in the correct plane!

Let us now study some photographs taken during live surgeries which illustrate the problems one can encounter when the anatomy is distorted and vital structures cannot be identified easily, and the dissection techniques one must follow in order to proceed further. The description is in third person and present continuous. The directions mentioned in the description, for example-the arrow pointing to the right shows-, the arrow pointing down shows-, etc. is with respect to the photograph and not with respect to the anatomy of the patient being operated. This is because the photographs have been taken from an angle that provided the best view and clarity during surgery.

Fundamental Precautions While Doing Hysterectomy (Fig. 3.1a–f)

1. The specimen, the uterus, is held with clamps applied on both sides with the assistant giving moderate upward traction (Fig. 3.1a). The ureters being retroperitoneal structures will tend to fall down as the specimen is pulled up by the assistant. The second assistant is retracting the bladder with help of Deaver's retractor. Both the round ligaments have been divided and a stay suture has been applied. On the left side, the tip of the artery forceps can be seen holding the

Fig. 3.1a

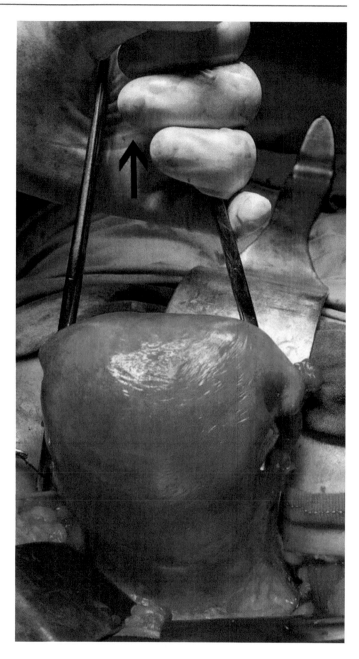

stay suture of the left round ligament. On the right side, one might be able to appreciate the rectus muscle has been partially divided transversely to facilitate better exposure.

2. Applying clamps as close as possible to the specimen (Fig. 3.1b) —one can see, the infundibulopelvic ligament has been clamped as close as possible to the ovary. The medial most clamp has been applied just along the ovarian margin, and a stout artery forceps has been applied between the two clamps. Now the infundibulopelvic ligament will be cut between the medical clamp and the artery forceps.

It is safer to first tie the cut infundibulopelvic ligament with a free tie before taking a transfixing suture medial to the free tie. This is because, sometimes, the tissues are very thin

Fig. 3.1b

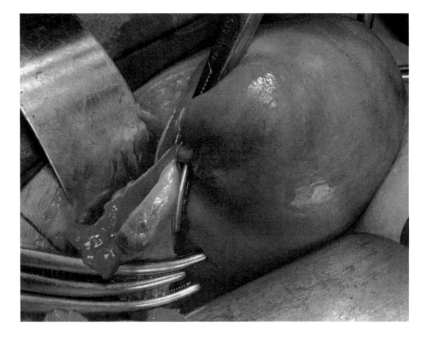

and friable. A stitch through a friable tissue will cut through, and if the clamps slip, it will lead to torrential hemorrhage. Remember, the ovarian artery which is present in the infundibulopelvic ligament is a direct branch of the descending aorta. Should the clamps slip, the artery will retract, and it may not be easy to locate the cut end of the bleeding artery. It might also require extending the incision or converting the laparoscopy to laparotomy. The ureters can be located very close to the infundibulopelvic ligament, and this is a common site where the ureter gets injured. Blind and hurried attempts to secure hemostasis, is the commonest cause of ureteric injuries.

Another reason for applying a free tie before transfixing the infundibulopelvic ligaments is that, if the needle pricks a vessel in the pedicle and if a hematoma occurs as a result, its extension is limited by the free tie which has already been applied. Some

gynecologists do not transfix the infundibulopelvic ligament at all. They just double ligate the infundibulopelvic ligament.

Throughout the surgery, the surgeon holds the pedicles while cutting and taking stitches. The first assistant holds the specimen with one hand and releases the clamps/cuts the sutures with the other. The second assistant facilitates exposure by holding the retractors as required and suctions out the cautery smoke and collected blood/fluid.

The assistant cauterizes the bleeders which have been held by the surgeon only after the surgeon has given the signal by saying "Touch." This is to avoid cauterizing any other tissue which may have been held by the forceps. The surgeon should also specify if cautery should be applied only as "touch and go," especially near vital structures like the bowel, ureter, base of bladder, etc. The assistant should also check if any metal structure is in contact with the cautery current

Fig. 3.1c

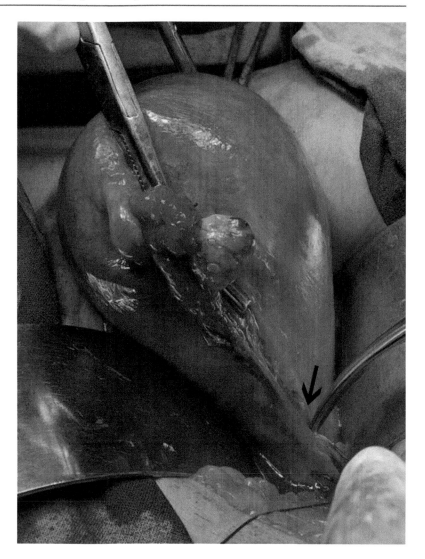

before cauterizing; because if this happens, it will lead to extensive burns and possibly catastrophic damage.

3. After the uterovesical fold has been excised, and the bladder pushed down, incise the posterior peritoneum of the uterus as well (Fig. 3.1c). This step is called the "skeletonization" of the uterine artery. The tortuous uterine artery can be seen after this step has been accomplished.

This is another important step which helps to prevent ureteric injury. The ureter being retroperitoneal falls lower down once the posterior peritoneum of the uterus has been incised and released.

4. Both, the uterovesical fold of peritoneum and the posterior peritoneum have been incised (Fig. 3.1d). Skeletonization of the uterine artery has been done. The uterine vessels can be seen at the level of the

Fig. 3.1d

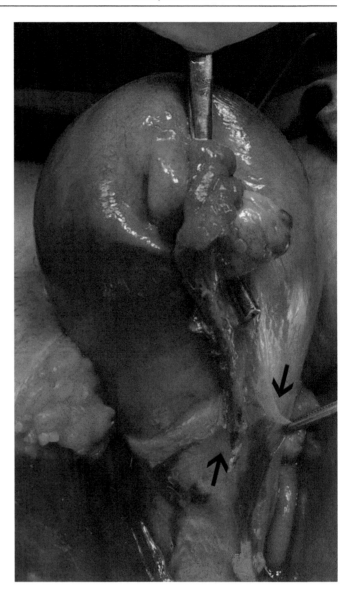

isthmus as shown by arrow pointing up. The uterine artery has a descending cervical branch and the upper branch anastomoses with the uterine branch of ovarian artery in the mesosalpinx.

Uterine clamps can now safely be applied; the ureters are very much down below. One can be sure that only the uterine vessels will be included in the clamp.

Skeletonization should not be skipped due to fear that it will cause "more bleeding" or that "so much of dissection" is not necessary. Small bleeders can be held with a fine tip forceps and cauterized, making sure that only the bleeding point is held and that there is no

Fig. 3.1e

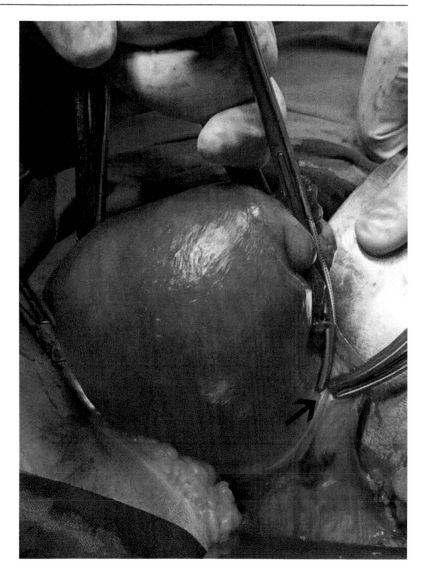

vital structure close to the held tissue. In Fig. 3.1d, one bleeding vessel on the anterior isthmus has been cauterized close to the specimen as shown by the cautery burn mark. The bladder has been pushed done and away from the operating field. And there is a bleeding vessel medial to the burn mark which needs to be cauterized. The spurt of bleeding can be appreciated. The arrow pointing down shows the posterior peritoneum. And one can see some bleeding is present along the cut margin of the peritoneum.

5. Uterine artery is clamped after skeletonization (Fig. 3.1e). The bladder has been pushed well below. The clamps have been applied at the level of the isthmus, as close to the specimen as possible, preferably by "overriding" the cervix. But this may not be

Fig. 3.1f

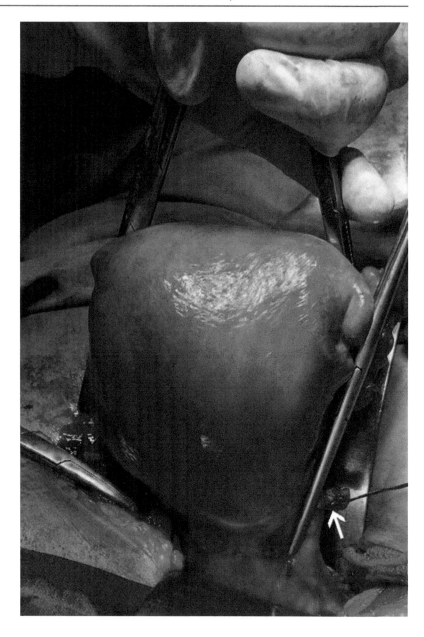

possible if the cervix is necrotic as in cases of a large endocervical fibroid with secondary infection.

6. All the subsequent clamps are applied medial to the previous pedicle (Fig. 3.1f). One can see the uterine artery has been clamped, cut, and ligated. The uterosacral clamp has been applied medial to the uterine artery pedicle. The arrow is pointing to the uterine artery pedicle. It is not advisable to keep a stay suture over the uterine artery or any vascular pedicle. Constant pulling of the stay suture can lead to the suture coming out or becoming loose—both will lead to hemorrhage which can manifest after the abdominal closure has been done. But in Fig. 3.1f, the uterine suture has been held temporarily for the purpose of taking the photograph—to make sure that the uterosacral clamp is applied medially and not lateral to it.

Bowel Dissection (Fig. 3.2, 3.3, 3.4, 3.5, 3.6, 3.7, 3.8, 3.9, 3.10, 3.11, 3.12, 3.13, 3.14, 3.15, 3.16 and 3.17)

One can see the loop of small intestine adherent to the lower part of the anterior abdominal wall above where the Allis forceps has been applied (Fig. 3.2a). Care has to be taken while opening the peritoneum. Carelessness while opening the peritoneum can lead to a bowel rent, which may be quite big requiring a major repair procedure.

Figure 3.2b is the close up view of the same case, i.e. Fig. 3.2a. Sharp dissection is being done using tissue cutting scissors. Never try to peel off/separate well-organized adhesions with a peanut or with wet or dry gauze. The arrow is pointing to the plane from where the dissection can begin.

Small intestine adherent to the anterior abdominal wall just below the level of umbilicus (Fig. 3.3)—if laparoscopy was planned, imagine the damage that would have occurred while inserting a Veress needle or during direct trocar insertion. An open method of inserting the camera port is safer, though not foolproof. The subsequent ports should be inserted under direct vision

taking care that instruments do not end up crossing each other.

So how does one open the peritoneum when one bowel is adherent to the overlying parietal peritoneum (Fig. 3.4a)?

The parietal peritoneum is held with two artery forceps, and felt with thumb and index finger (Fig. 3.4b). After ensuring that there is no structure underneath, a small opening is made with a sharp instrument and then the peritoneal opening is extended in the direction where there is no adherent structure. After the opening is large enough to permit adequate visualization, the bowel loops can be released from the overlying parietal peritoneum. This step is important even if the patient has no symptoms relating to bowels because postoperative adhesions can make any possible future surgery more difficult and can also cause subacute intestinal obstruction in future. Releasing all the bowel adhesions during the present surgery will also enable the gynecologist to pack the bowels away from the operating field and reduce chances of bowel injury.

The peritoneum has been opened, but there is still an adherent loop to the anterior abdominal wall (Fig. 3.4c). One can appreciate the bowel

Fig. 3.2a

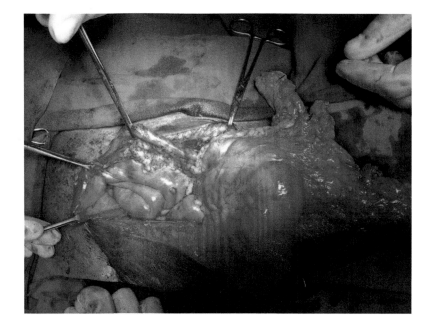

Fig. 3.2b

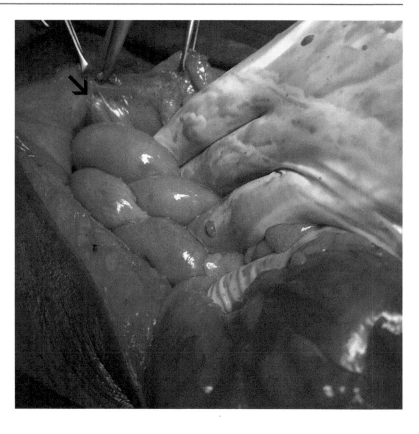

Fig. 3.3

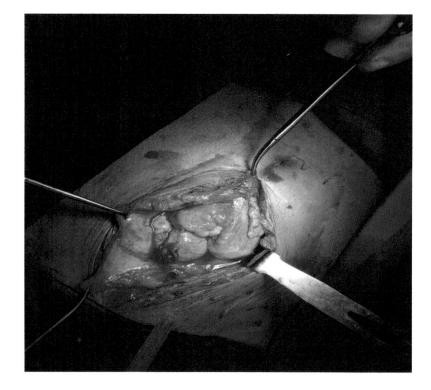

Fig. 3.4a

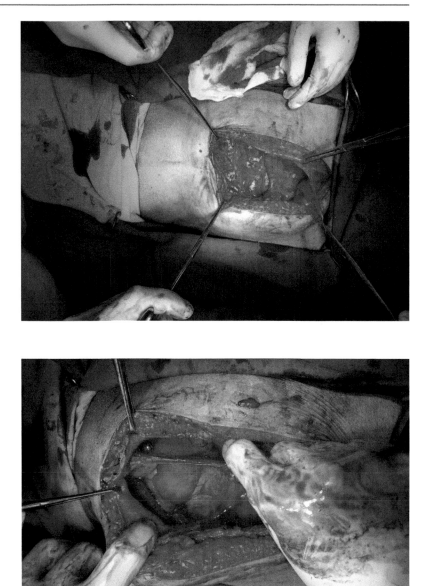

Fig. 3.4b

loops inside; they are agglutinated to one another. Extensive dissection will now have to be performed.

A part of parietal peritoneum has been excised to release the loop of bowel from the anterior abdominal wall (Fig. 3.5). Now using sharp dissection, the loops will have to be separated.

Sharp dissection using tissue cutting scissors should be done to separate the adherent bowel loops (Fig. 3.6). Counter traction by the assistant is showing the plane along which the dissection can be done. The suction cannula is pointing to the plane in which the bowel loops can be separated.

Fig. 3.4c

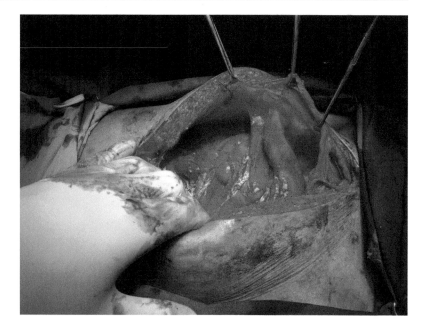

Fig. 3.5

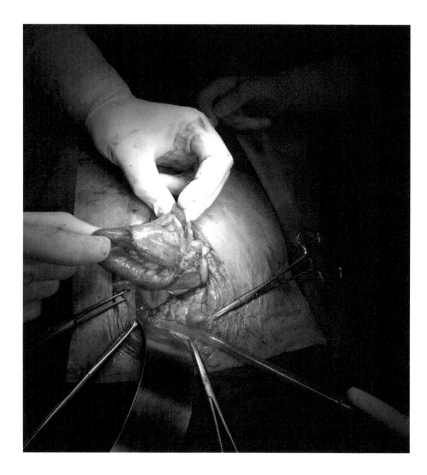

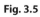

Fig. 3.6

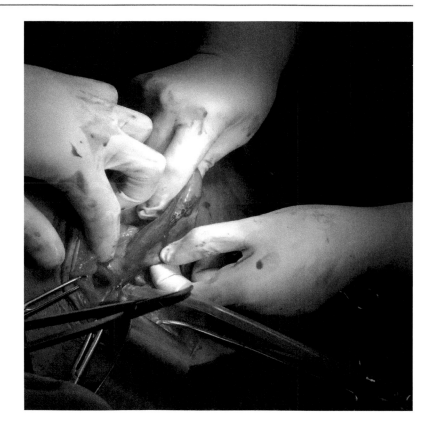

A segment of small intestine is adherent to the dome of bladder (Fig. 3.7). The surgeon must feel the bulb of the Foley catheter to confirm the bladder location. One must check for possible bladder injury before closure; is there any watery fluid filling the pelvis, or is the tip of Foley catheter seen. Retrograde filling with methylene blue-stained saline can be done. A urologist must be called if the injury is in the trigone or the posterior bladder wall.

Sometimes bowel loops are densely adherent to the vaginal vault following hysterectomy (Fig. 3.8), the ovary, seen as pearly white/grayish white structure, can be well appreciated. It is behind the adherent loop of small intestine.

Adhesions between folds of mesentery (Fig. 3.9)—this is preventing the gynecologist from getting a full exposure of the pelvis. One will have to separate them before proceeding fur-ther. Trying to pack the bowel without releasing these adhesions can damage the bowel and can cause mesenteric tears. Vertical rent in the mesentery does not cut off blood supply to the bowel. Transverse rents in the mesentery can cut off the blood supply to the affected bowel segment.

At the end of the surgery, it would be advisable to explore the entire length of the bowel. Check if there are any purplish patches over any of the bowel segments. Suture the rents in the mesentery to prevent internal herniation. If there is any damage, call a surgeon. It is better to discover such injuries on table than a few hours later when the patient is in the postoperative recovery room.

A panoramic view of showing adhesions between bowel loop and mesentery (Fig. 3.10); it would be advisable to separate such adhesions even if they are not causing any symptoms for

Fig. 3.7

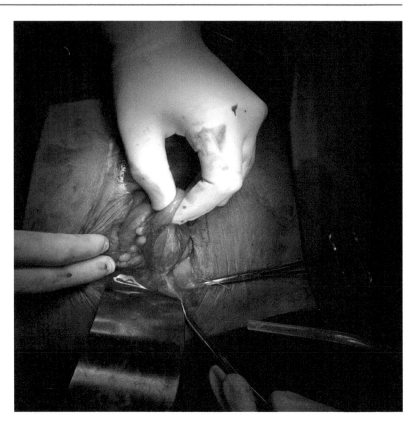

Fig. 3.8

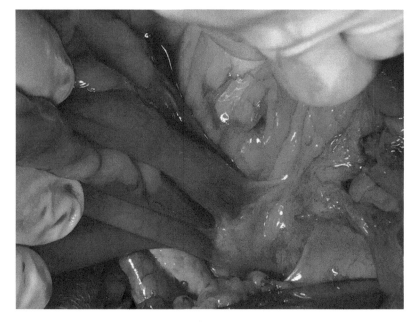

Fig. 3.9

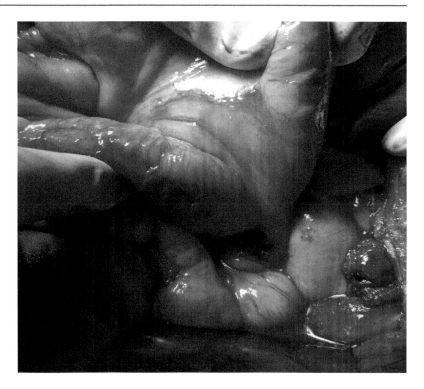

Fig. 3.10

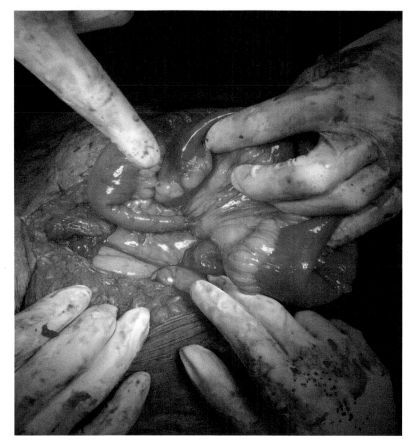

two reasons. First, they prevent the operating gynecologist from entering the pelvis, where the gynecological pathology lies. Trying to operate without getting full exposure will only increase the chances of injuries because of extensive handling and retraction. Second, these adhesions will get organized further and eventually cause intestinal obstruction (subacute or acute) for which the patient may have to get operated once again [7, 8]. In case of subacute presentation, the diagnosis might get postponed for long periods because the patient might assume that she has age-related "weakening" of digestion. She might acclimatize herself by having small meals consisting of semisolid food. The patient might end up losing a lot of weight and may have poor nutritional status at the time of surgery.

A panoramic view of the entire small intestine after adhesiolysis (Fig. 3.11a–c).

Fortunately, there is no bowel injury (Fig. 3.11a). The small intestine is pink throughout its length.

Now that the small intestine has been freed (Fig. 3.11b), the gynecologist can enter the pelvis, but there is something on closer inspection—more adhesions?

Close-up view showing the entire small intestine exposed after adhesiolysis (Fig. 3.11c); the intestines are pink in color with no bluish-purplish patches, suggesting that the blood supply is intact and the mesentery has not been damaged. However, there are quite a few flimsy adhesions between bowel loops as shown by the arrow. They will have to be separated, otherwise they can cause intestinal obstruction once they become organized.

The pelvic structures are now exposed, and the gynecological aspect of the surgery will now begin.

Fig. 3.11a

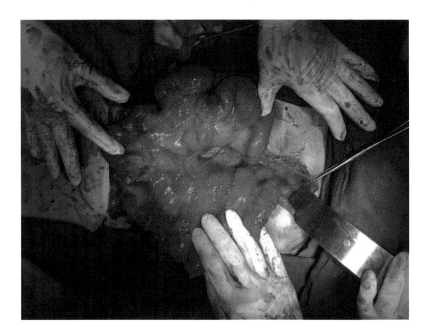

Fig. 3.11b

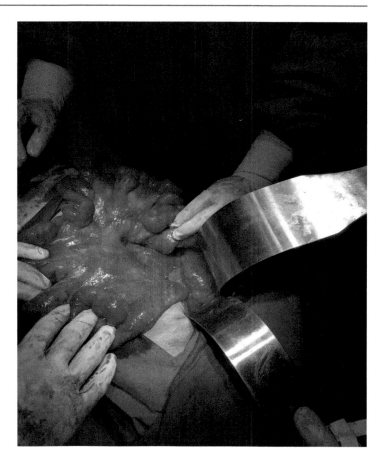

Fig. 3.11c

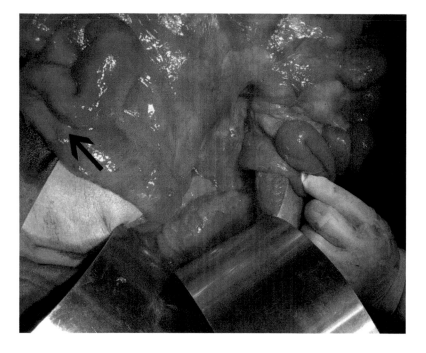

Can Bowel Adhesions Present as a Case of Adnexal Mass!?
(Fig. 3.12a–e)

The upper bowel adhesions have been divided, and the access to the pelvis has been achieved (Fig. 3.12a). But the pelvic organs are not quite made out. Is the loop of bowel which is stuck inside the pelvis, the small or large intestine? Is that band seen on the bowel wall , the teniae coli? What is the pearly white structure in the right corner? Is it the ovary?

This patient presented with pain and had a large adnexal mass on imaging. She had undergone hysterectomy earlier. Whether the ovaries were removed during hysterectomy was not known, since there were no records.

But look a bit more closely (Fig. 3.12b). A close inspection of the case shows that the loop of bowel which is stuck to the right side of the pelvis

is the small intestine. The upper arrow is pointing to some bands, they ARE NOT teniae coli, the bands which distinguish the large intestine from the small intestine. Sometimes, unless one inspects the bowels carefully, one can end up confusing small intestine for the large intestine, or for that matter the dilated fallopian tube for a loop of intestine. One may have to dissect carefully to expose more of the structure in question. One has to confirm that the longitudinal band is teniae coli which are present along the "entire" length of large intestine, whereas a few adhesions can initially be mistaken for the teniae coli, but will not run like a band throughout the length of the intestine.

The other arrow is pointing to a pearly white structure. Is it the ovary?

Another image from the same case (Fig. 3.12c), reveals no ovary. There is nothing to suggest as an adnexal mass, as indicated by

Fig. 3.12a

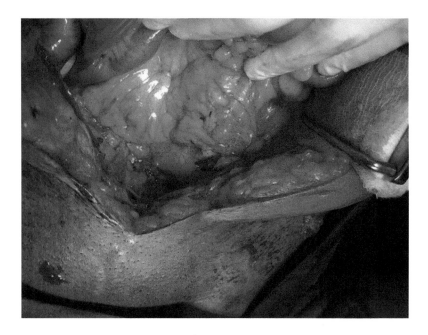

Fig. 3.12b

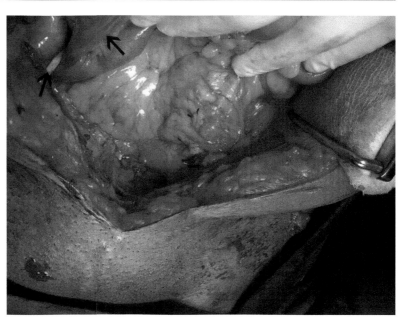

the CT scan either. Bowel is still adherent, and it will have to be released to give a clearer picture. The arrow pointing down is showing what looks like the mesentery. Or is it the appendices epiploicae? The arrow pointing to the right is showing vault adhesions which have formed after hysterectomy.

A close-up view showing the in situ pelvic findings (Fig. 3.12d); the Babcock's forceps is holding what seems to be fairly obvious as the appendix. The arrow pointing up is showing the caecum which is hidden under the small intestine. The small intestine with the mesentery is adherent to the pelvic structures, as indicated by the arrow pointing down. It is now also quite clear that the bands on the small intestine wall are what might be adhesion bands. They certainly are not teniae coli.

The white structure looks like the caecum (and it is not the ovary), it certainly is a structure with a lumen. After releasing the loop of adherent small intestine, one can confirm what that white structure is. The initial cursory look had given the impression that the loop of bowel stuck in the pelvis was the large intestine. But now it is clear, it is the small intestine.

Now the teniae coli of caecum have become a bit more obvious (Fig. 3.12e). After releasing the segment of small intestine from the vault, it will be clear as to what the pathology is.

After releasing all the adhesions, it is now obvious that there is no adnexal mass (Fig. 3.12f). The patient presented with abdominal pain, and the imaging showed a huge adnexal mass. The adnexal mass was actually bowel loops adherent to each other due to postoperative adhesions. There are no ovaries, they must have removed during hysterectomy. Adhesions due to previous surgery can present to a gynecologist as an adnexal mass.

Fig. 3.12c

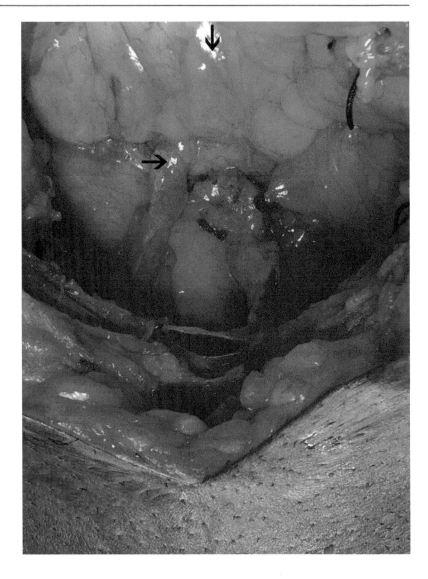

Fig. 3.12d

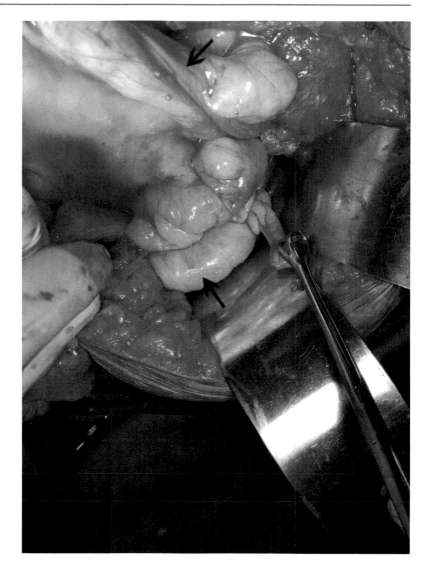

Fig. 3.12e

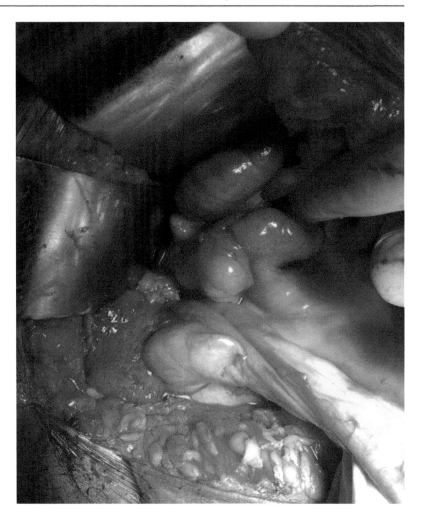

Fig. 3.12f

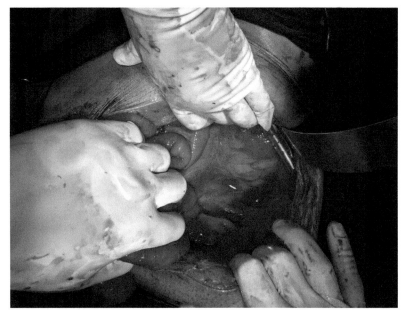

Uterus and the Ovaries Completely Buried Under Bowel Adhesions
(Figs. 3.13, 3.14a, b, 3.15a, b, 3.16a, b, and 3.17)

The fundus of the uterus has become visible after bowel adhesiolysis (Fig. 3.13), though a lot of adhesions are yet to be released. One can appreciate that the omentum had to be cut to expose the pelvis. The stump of the cut omentum (with silk ligature) is seen below the upper Deaver's retractors.

The structure on the left side of the image just above the lower Deaver's retractor looks like the ovary, or is it the large intestine (Fig. 3.13)? One cannot be sure till all the adhesions are released.

The ovary has become visible only after adhesiolysis (Fig. 3.14a). It looks benign, but try to remove it without causing rupture or intraoperative spillage. Only the final histopathology report will confirm the benign, borderline, or malignant nature of the tumor. If it is early malignancy, an intraoperative spillage will upstage it to stage I C. Therefore, use sharp dissection to separate the ovary which is densely adherent to adjacent structures. Avoid plucking it out, though it might be tempting.

Figure 3.14b is another image from the previous case—the ovary is now easy to resect, with most adhesions having been separated. One can appreciate the thick patch of fibrous adhesions of the surface. The capsule is intact and there is no spillage.

The mesentery is adherent to what appears like an ovarian tumor (Fig. 3.15a).

It is now obvious that it is indeed a case of an ovarian tumor (Fig. 3.15b).

Ovaries identified at last (Fig. 3.16a).

This is an example of a patient in whom carcinoma cervix was detected following abdominal hysterectomy a couple of years ago. She had received radiation following hysterectomy. She presented with chronic pain abdomen, and the pelvic examination showed tenderness in the adnexa.

After menopause, the levels of gonadotropins increase permanently, and this can cause

Fig. 3.13

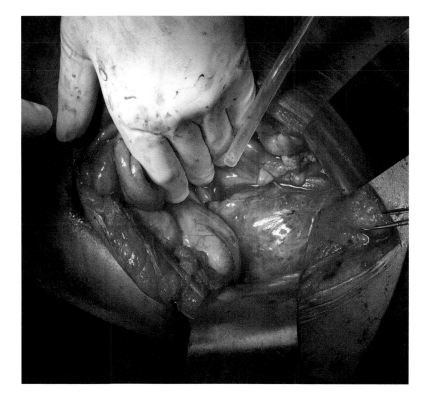

Fig. 3.14a

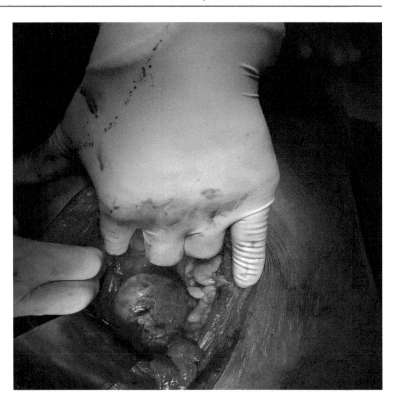

Fig. 3.14b

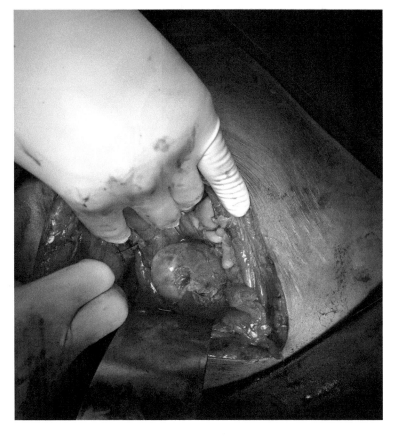

Fig. 3.15a

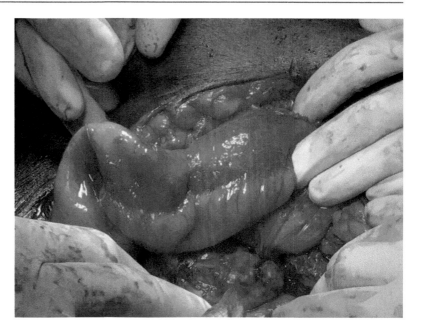

Fig. 3.15b

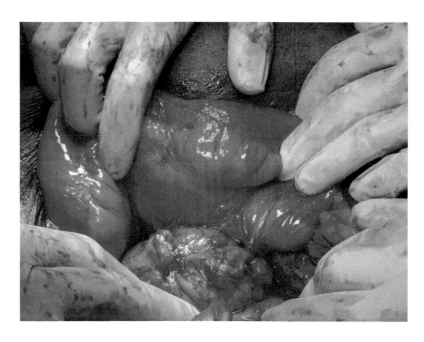

Fig. 3.16a

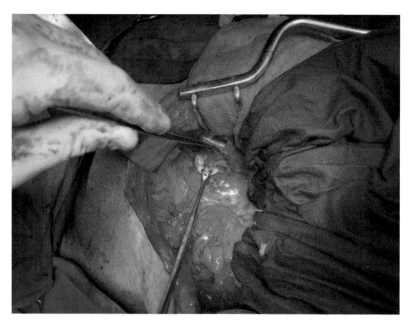

Fig. 3.16b

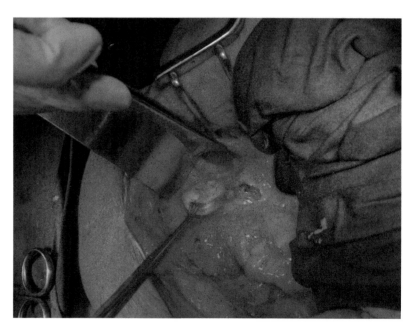

problems like hirsutism [9]. This is due to the fact that under the influence of raised gonadotropin levels, the stroma of the postmenopausal ovaries secretes increased levels of androgens. Apart from being a cosmetic problem, this can increase the risk of cardiovascular diseases because increased levels of androgens worsen the lipid profile.

Any remnant of ovarian tissue inadvertently left behind can also enlarge under the influence of raised postmenopausal gonadotropins and cause symptoms like pain.

In this patient, the symptoms were probably due to adhesions.

The ovary is now on the verge of being removed (Fig. 3.16b). The inverted end of the

Fig. 3.17

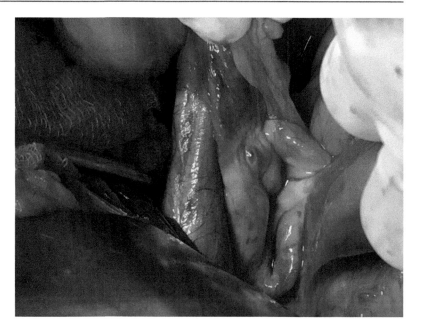

tissue forceps is exposing the retroperitoneal space. The ureter seems to be quite down and away from the areas of dissection. Previous radiation has made opening of spaces difficult. Any forced opening of spaces can lead to the blood vessels; especially the veins getting torn and can lead to torrential bleeding. It will then be very difficult to locate the internal iliac artery for ligation. Moreover, if the veins are damaged, a vascular surgeon will have to be called without any further delay, and it will not be easy for him either!

Another example of an atrophic ovary adherent to the intestine (right side of the image) and the peritoneum of the lateral pelvic wall (Fig. 3.17); to excise the ovary, one has to do sharp dissection. Hold the bleeding points with a fine tip forceps and lift it away from the underlying structure, that is, make sure that the underlying bowel/bladder/ureter are well away and then cauterize. Remember that the thermal damage due to cautery extends well beyond the visible area of charring. The charred patch on the bowel/bladder/ureter might slough away over the next few days and will present as a bowel perforation/vesicovaginal fistula/ureterovaginal fistula, usually a week after the surgery.

Can an Ovarian Mass Grow Retroperitoneally? (Fig. 3.18a–d)

A lady who was admitted for fever was incidently found to have a very big asymptomatic adnexal mass. She had undergone abdominal hysterectomy a couple of years back. She has no symptoms related to the mass and on examination, she had nothing to suggest the presence of an adnexal mass. Tumor markers were normal. She was posted for surgery when she recovered from fever. On table, no mass was found in the pelvis. However, careful examination shows that there is something in the retroperitoneum (Fig. 3.18a).

Further dissection shows a cystic mass hidden behind the sigmoid (Fig. 3.18b). The teniae coli of the sigmoid are obvious.

The mass is now exposed (Fig. 3.18c). Care has to be taken not to dissect the sigmoid in such a way that the mesosigmoid gets trimmed away from the sigmoid. That would be a disastrous situation. The upper limit of the cyst is till the splenic flexure. One cannot try to remove through a small incision; the incision has to be extended lest the large bowel gets damaged.

Fig. 3.18a

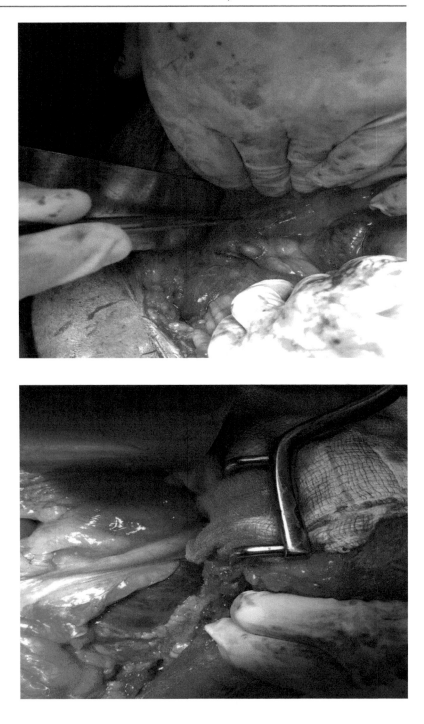

Fig. 3.18b

The same case being viewed from the opposite side (Fig. 3.18d); the sigmoid is being pushed down by the assistant's fingers, and the surgeon is holding the small intestine.

The histopathology revealed an "Endometriotic cyst"!

Bowel Mass? Or is it an Ovarian Mass? (Fig. 3.19a, b)

An adnexal mass which is adherent more to the sigmoid than to the uterus (Fig. 3.19a, b).

Fig. 3.18c

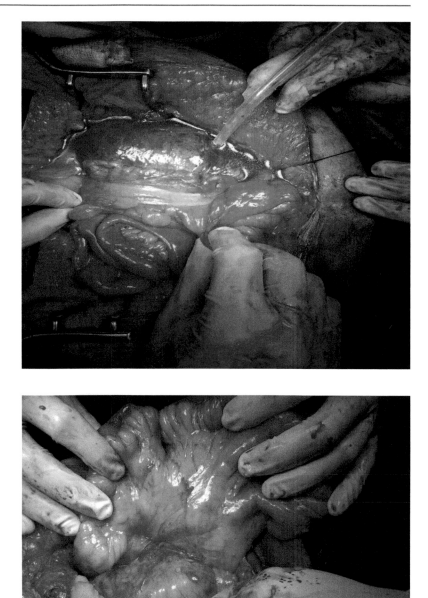

Fig. 3.18d

There is a large pelvic mass, but is it a gynecological condition or something to do with the bowel (Fig. 3.19a)? The arrow is pointing toward the teniae coli. It is obvious at this point that it is the large intestine. But the demarcation between the mass and the bowel wall is not obvious. So careful sharp dissection has to be done lest portion of the large intestine is also removed along with the mass. The gynecologist has to check time and again while separating the adnexal mass from sigmoid. Is the mesosigmoid is being cut? Is the blood supply of the sigmoid is being stripped off?

Fig. 3.19a

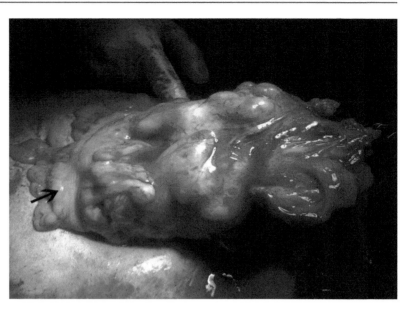

Fig. 3.19b

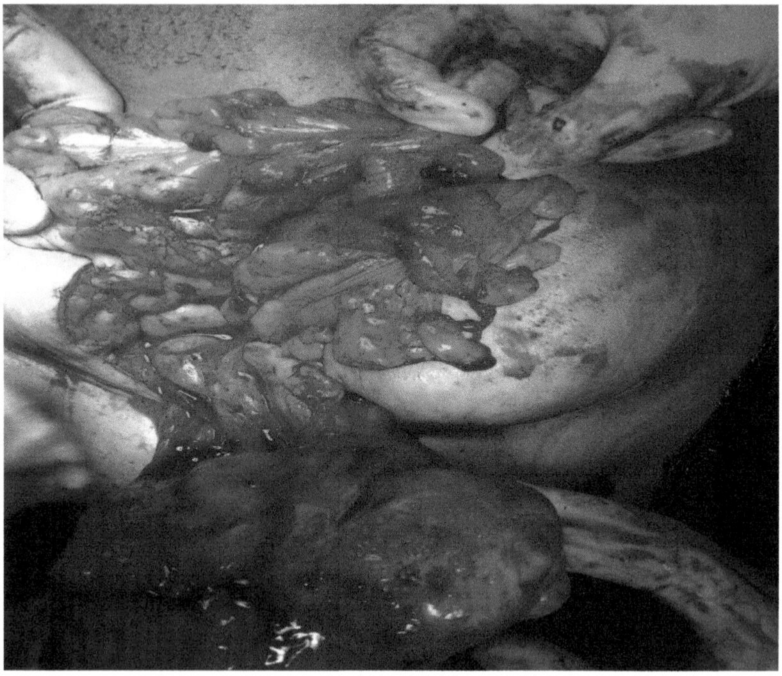

Using sharp dissection, the mass has been separated (Fig. 3.19b). From the gross appearance of the mass, it is clear that it is fleshy, and is likely to be gynecological in origin. Note the color of the sigmoid. It is pink and healthy. The blood supply has not been stripped off. The adnexal mass looks like a leiomyoma, on gross examination. But remember, a very fleshy vascular leiomyoma which may have suddenly increased in size in recent past may be a sarcoma/sarcomatous transformation of a preexisting leiomyoma. Avoid excising/removing the leiomyoma piecemeal. Intraoperative spillage can upstage what could be an early stage malignancy. Uterine sarcomas are notorious for recurrence, despite adjuvant chemotherapy [10].

How to Locate the Ureter in a Usual Case?

To locate the ureter transperitonealy (Fig. 3.20a–c).

1. The pouch of Douglas (Fig. 3.20a).

   Ureters can be seen transperitoneally, if there are no adhesions or color changes (due to endometriosis).

   This image has been taken during LSCS. The baby has been delivered, and the uterus has been closed. One can appreciate the congested ovarian vessels.

2. To locate the ureters transperitoneally, expose the either side of the pouch of Douglas (Fig. 3.20b). The rectum has been depressed with the first assistant's hands, and the second assistant is holding the fundus. The uterus has been exteriorized.

   One can see the ureter crossing the bifurcation of the common iliac artery. This is better appreciated during LSCS when tissue edema helps in better visualization and the planes easier to separate.

3. A close-up view—here one can appreciate the bifurcation of the common iliac artery as shown by arrow pointing left (Fig. 3.20c). The external iliac artery can be seen running a straight course down as shown by the arrow pointing up. On careful examination, one can see a tubular structure as shown by the arrow pointing to the right. This is the ureter. One might be able to appreciate its crossing the bifurcation of the common iliac artery. One can gently stimulate the ureter, transperitoneally with a blunt forceps to look for peristalsis.

Fig. 3.20a

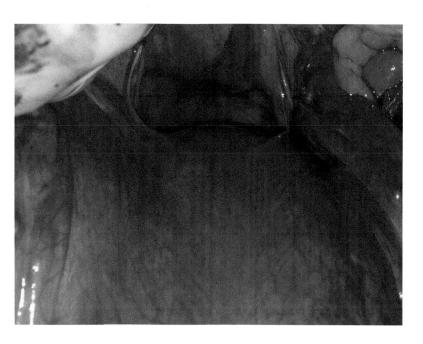

Fig. 3.20b

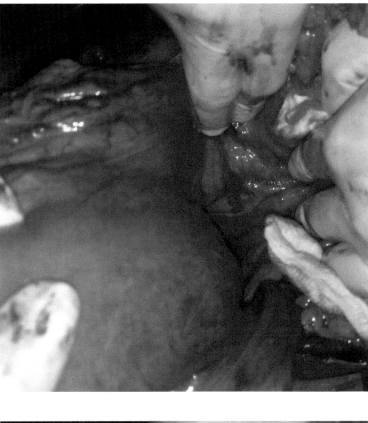

Fig. 3.20c

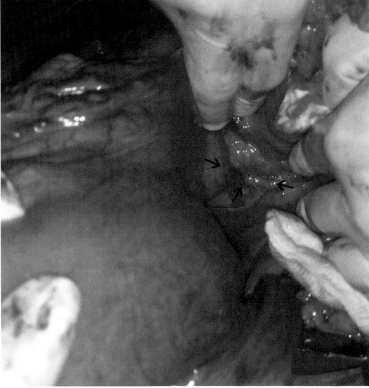

How to Expose the Ureter
(Fig. 3.21a–i)

1. Divide the round ligament (Fig. 3.21a). The round ligament is the most consistent landmark in the female pelvis. Apply a stay suture after dividing it.

2. Hold the round ligament with two clamps (Fig. 3.21b). In this image one can see that there is a well-circumscribed ovarian mass.

3. The round ligament has been divided and a stay suture has been applied on the lateral cut end (Fig. 3.21c). The two folds of the broad ligament have been opened. Now the loose

Fig. 3.21a

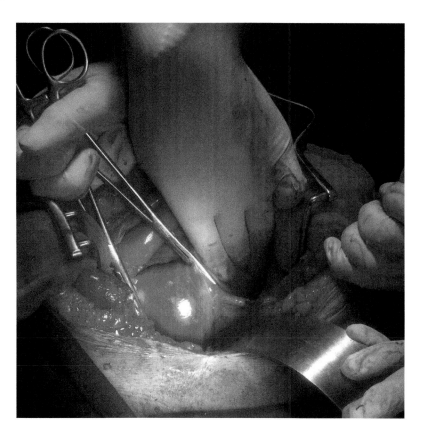

Fig. 3.21b

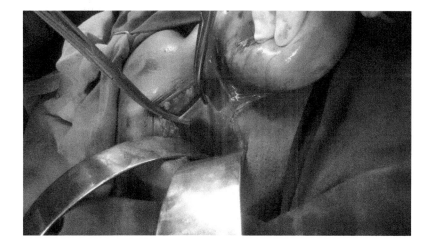

Fig. 3.21c

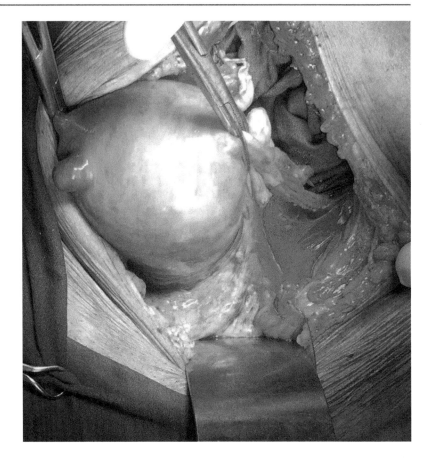

areolar tissue will be separated to visualize the underlying structures. One can do blunt dissection with fingers in this case since the planes are easily separable.

4. After the broad ligament has been opened, the loose areolar tissue has been cleared (Fig. 3.21d). The "axilla" of the pelvis has been exposed. Now, one has to locate the bifurcation of common iliac artery, the external iliac artery, and the internal iliac artery. The ureter will be seen crossing the bifurcation of common iliac artery. Ureter will show peristalsis when stimulated by a blunt instrument, whereas the arteries will be seen pulsating.

5. Arrow 1 shows the obliterated umbilical artery (Fig. 3.21e). The anterior division of the internal iliac divides into the following branches in a female pelvis: superior vesical, inferior vesical, inferior gluteal, uterine, obturator, internal pudendal, and middle rectal arteries. It then continues as the obliterated umbilical artery as shown by arrow 1. Arrow 2 shows the external iliac artery which runs a straight course and passes under the inguinal ligament to continue as the femoral artery. The blue structure below the external iliac artery is the external iliac vein.

Should the external iliac artery be ligated instead of the internal iliac artery to control pelvic hemorrhage, lower limb pulse and ischemic necrosis of the lower limb will be absent. Check for femoral pulses after ligating the internal iliac artery to be doubly sure.

Fig. 3.21d

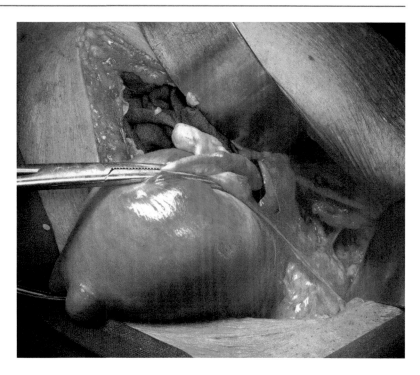

Fig. 3.21e

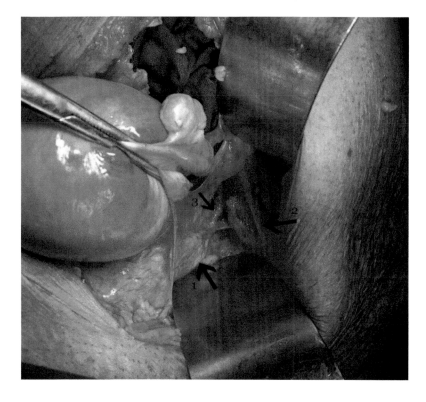

Arrow 3 is pointing at the internal iliac artery. If we go higher up, we will find the bifurcation of the common iliac artery.

So where is the ureter in the image above? Ureter can be felt running medially along the leaf of the broad ligament. If one sees the image carefully, one can appreciate a tubular structure just below the number "3." That appears to be the ureter. Just feel it with your thumb and index finger. If it feels like a cord that slips between your fingers, then it is the ureter. The tactile feel will be the same in every case. It will never vary from patient to patient, like the feel of a leiomyoma, which can be soft if necrotic due to torsion, hard if calcified, and firm in most cases.

The texture of an organ can vary from patient to patient. For example, intestines can feel soft and friable if there is a lot of inflammation due to pus and peritonitis,

pale and like lead pipe after radiation, and distended or collapsed depending on the amount of gas. Similarly, the fallopian tube can feel calcified or soft depending on the condition. The feel of the uterus can be hard if there are calcified leiomyomas, soft and fleshy in case of a sarcoma; even a gravid uterus can feel woody hard in case of abruptio placentae. But the feel of the ureter will always be like a cord that slips between fingers. Once experienced, this sensation will not be forgotten.

6. Another view from the previous case (Fig. 3.21f) showing the ureter is seen along the fold of broad ligament. It has crossed the bifurcation of common iliac artery. It will now pass under the uterine artery lower down its course. The external iliac artery running straight down continues as the femoral artery in the lower limb, and the internal iliac artery

Fig. 3.21f

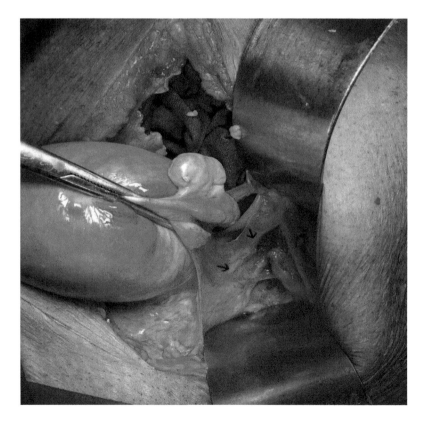

Fig. 3.21g

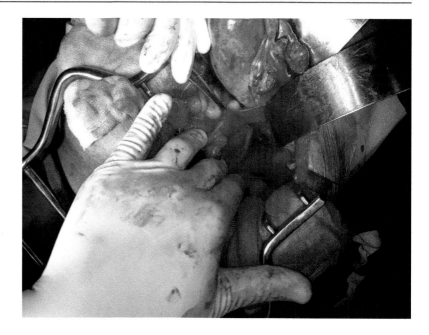

can also be well appreciated. If one gently dissects the areolar tissues along the course of ureter, one can find the "water under the bridge"—the ureter coursing below the uterine artery which is a branch of the anterior division of the internal iliac artery.

7. The ureter has been exposed well (Fig. 3.21g). The areolar tissue above it has been dissected, and now it is seen very clearly. Sometimes it may not be possible to expose it so clearly due to induration and fibrosis. In such situations, one can try to locate it with fingers and confirm by feeling a cord that slips between fingers. This should be done before applying clamps and cutting, or taking deep stitches, or cauterizing blindly. Remember that the pelvic part of the ureter is its least vascular segment, and if the injury is detected on table (a better situation to be in, than discovering it a week later due to the formation of ureterovaginal fistula), it will require extensive repair and not just a simple ureteroureterostomy. Complete transection or ligation of the ureter presents as reduced urine output and severe flank pain in the immediate postoperative period.

Injury of any kind to the ureter will require a urologist and possibly extensive repair.

8. The arrow is pointing toward the ureter (Fig. 3.21h). One Deaver's retractor (the lower one) is inserted just above the pubic symphysis. The other Deaver's retractor is inserted into the retroperitoneal space. The rectum is seen and pushed behind by the surgeon's fingers, and the infundibulopelvic ligament has been ligated and cut.

9. Now that the ureter has been visualized (Fig. 3.21i), as shown by the arrow, apply clamps and cut the infundibulopelvic ligament without any doubt or hesitation. And in case one cannot visualize, then feel it with the thumb and index fingers before applying clamps and cutting. This step is essential in preventing ureteric injuries in cases of large ovarian tumors/adnexal masses.

Fig. 3.21h

Fig. 3.21i

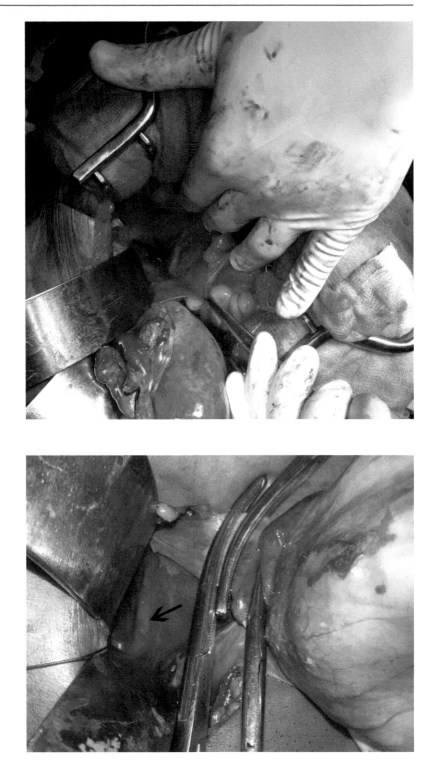

How to Confirm the Location of the Ureter if There is a Lot of Fibrosis/Oozing/Planes not Well Demarcated (Figs. 3.22a–c, 3.23, 3.24, and 3.25a, b)?

1. Gentle dissection is the first rule. Do not forcefully try to open any space. One can appreciate the oozing in the retroperitoneal space (Fig. 3.33a). Do not apply cautery indiscriminately.

   The Deavor retractor is exposing the retroperitoneal space (Fig. 3.22a). The tip of suction cannula is being used to remove all the oozing blood from the operating field. The ureter must be located somewhere there.

2. Hold the bleeding vessels with a fine tip/vascular forceps and cauterize them (Fig. 3.22b). Make sure that no other structure is held and the metal forceps is not touching any other structure. Check the cautery current. Avoid cautery burns and injuries. The last thing that anybody would want is a ureteric stricture or a fistula showing up after 5 days! Figure 3.22b shows the uterine artery which has been ligated and cut. One can see the two silk ligatures. The ureter is seen emerging from below the lower stump of the uterine artery.

3. Gentle sharp dissection; do a little at a time. The reason for induration and a plane not being well formed is now obvious (Fig. 3.22c).

There is a bead of pus (seen right adjacent to fine tip forceps). But do not force open the space with finger or any instrument. The presence of pus means that the iliac vessels, especially the veins which are thin walled, are friable and can be easily torn off leading to torrential hemorrhage.

4. Do not traumatize any structure with rough suctioning (Fig. 3.23). When there is inflammation, expect the vessel walls, especially the veins to be thin and friable; even suctioning can traumatize the vessels and can cause torrential bleeding. Try and palpate the ureter. Go ahead with sharp dissection once the location of the ureter is confirmed and that it is away from the operating field. The forceps is pointing the external iliac artery (Fig. 3.23). The clipped pubic hair can be seen which indicates which side is the lower end of the incision. One can also see cautery burn marks to the right of the fine tip forceps. The cautery burn marks are pinpoint and well above and not involving the serosa of the artery. The arrow is pointing at the fat and areolar tissue along the fold of broad ligament. The ureter must be somewhere here. The internal iliac artery is seen underneath. At the level of ischial spine, the ureter will take a sharp medial turn and enter the tunnel of Wertheim passing under the uterine artery, a branch of anterior division of the internal iliac artery.

Fig. 3.22a

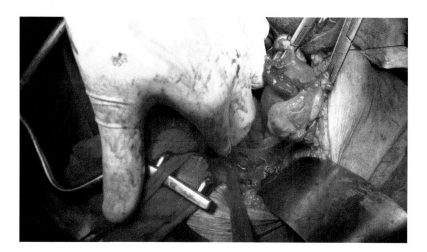

Fig. 3.22b

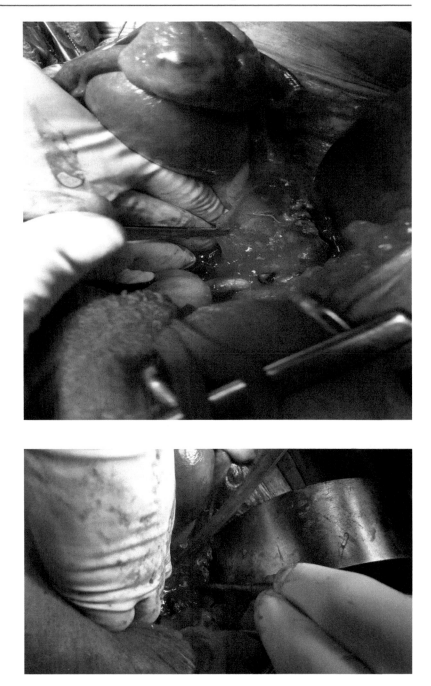

Fig. 3.22c

5. Bleeding is bound to occur when there is a lot of induration. How to cauterize bleeding vessels in such situations? The ureter is located very close to the bleeding points. Indiscriminate use of cautery will lead to ureteric injuries.

   Hold only the bleeding point and cauterize it. Make sure there is nothing in the chunk of tissue that has been held. The image shows a bleeder that has been held over the psoas muscle (Fig. 3.24).

6. Tackling bleeding—the ureter has been exposed (Fig. 3.25a). The forceps is holding a fold of the broad ligament, just above the cautery burn mark. The cautery burn is well above the course of ureter, which is seen running downward. There is a stay suture over

Fig. 3.23

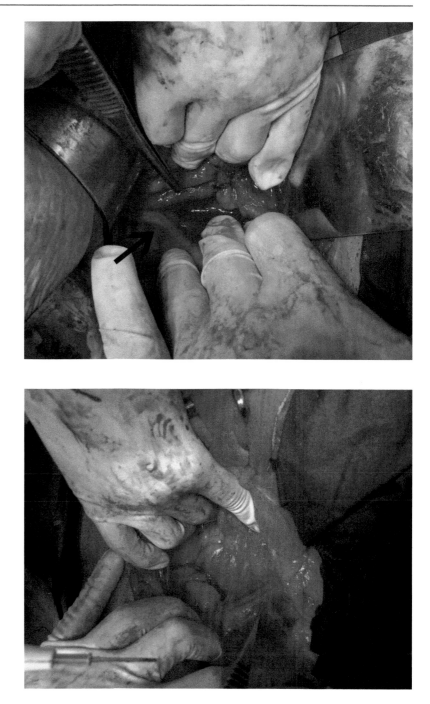

Fig. 3.24

the lateral cut end of the round ligament (which is not visible) on the left side of the image. The appendices epiploicae of the sigmoid are touching the forceps. So while one is cauterizing the bleeding vessels or taking a stitch, one must not only make sure that there is no other structure held in the forceps or the stitch but also see that the intestine behind the fold of broad ligament is well retracted and not in contact. Otherwise there can be a cautery burn on the bowel loop, or a portion of it can get included in the stitch.

7. A close-up view (Fig. 3.25b)—the arrow is pointing at the ureter which has been located

Fig. 3.25a

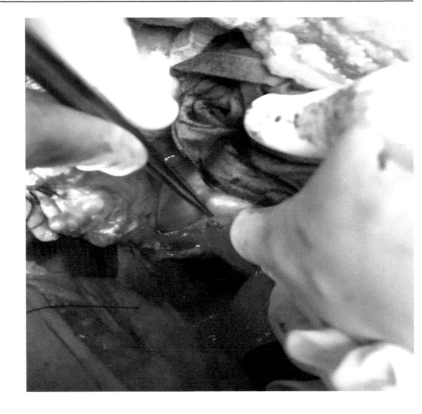

Fig. 3.25b

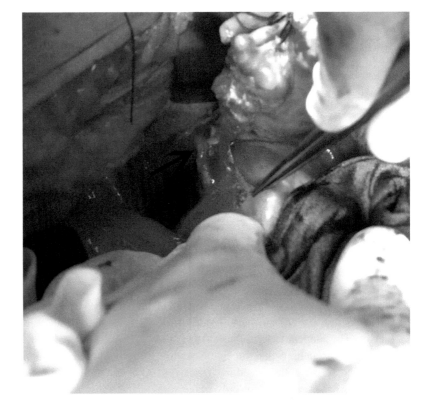

and is well away from the bleeding vessels. The bleeding vessels can now be held and cauterized, without the fear of ureter suffering cautery burns. But make sure the metal forceps is not touching any other structure, other than the bleeding points. In Fig. 3.25b, the appendices epiploicae of the sigmoid is in contact with the forceps. Push it down before the cautery current passes through the forceps.

How to Take Ureter on a Tape
(Fig. 3.26a–g)?

1. Expose the ureter first (Fig. 3.26a). If one has any doubts, then gently stimulate the structure with a blunt instrument. Ureter will show peristalsis, and arteries will be seen pulsating. Hold with thumb and index finger, and it will feel like a cord that slips.

2. Pass the right-angled forceps, also called mixter, under the ureter (Fig. 3.26b). For accomplishing this step, ask the assistant to expose the retroperitoneal space with Deaver's retractors. Hold the fold of the broad ligament with the left hand (if one is a right-hander), behind the ureter. Using the right-angled forceps in the right hand, gently dissect the areolar tissue below the ureter where it has been exposed and is best visible. Now, pass the tips of the business ends of the right-angled forceps below the ureter. Figure 3.26b shows a stay suture on the round ligament (which is not visible, it is buried under the Deaver's retractor). One can also see a clamp holding a chunk of tissue; lumens of the multiple cut vessels can also be seen in it).

3. In Fig, 3.26c, the arrow pointing down is showing the ureter with the right-angled forceps under it. The arrow pointing up is showing the cut uterine artery held by a clamp. Now it has to be ligated. The lumen of the cut artery can be appreciated. Now the assistant can feed a tape to the right-angled forceps, which can be taken out from below the ureter. This will result in the ureter being taken on a tape.

4. Now the tape has been passed under the ureter (Fig. 3.26d). Do not pull; just keep it on one side. This step goes a long way in lateralizing the ureter. In cases where there are dense adhesions, large adnexal masses, etc., this step helps in keeping the ureter away from the operating field and helps preventing injuries.

Fig. 3.26a

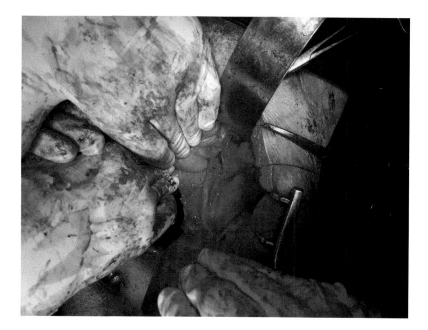

Fig. 3.26b

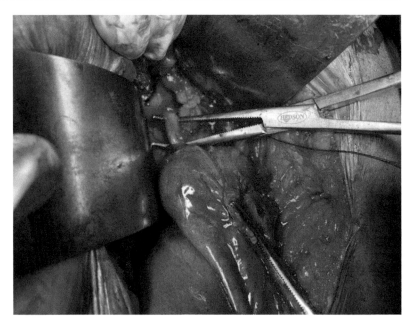

Fig. 3.26c

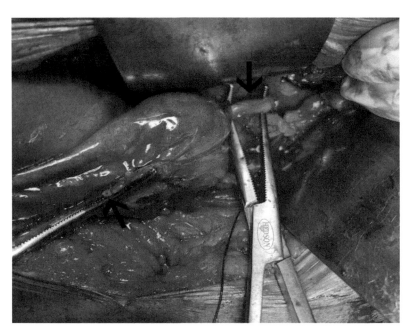

Make sure to keep a count of the tape before closing the abdomen!

5. In Fig. 3.26e, the horizontal arrow is showing the ureter which has been taken on a tape. The tape is soaked in blood, but it can be appreciated if one observes a bit carefully.

   The right-angled forceps is now under the uterine artery, as indicated by the arrow pointing up. A typical picture of "water under the bridge"; the ureter is seen passing under the uterine artery. The uterine artery is running medially to the isthmus of the uterus.

6. An example of planes not being well formed (Fig. 3.26f).

   At the upper end, one can see a part of the ureter that has been exposed and has

Fig. 3.26d

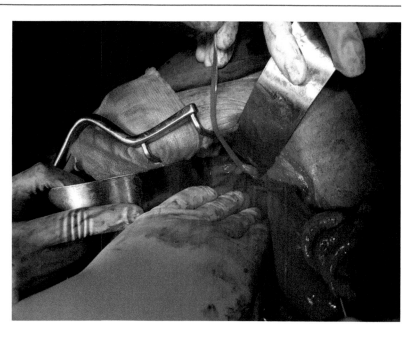

Fig. 3.26e

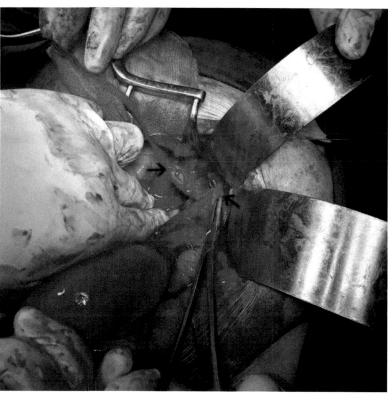

been taken on a tape (look above, just adjacent to the upper Deaver's retractor). The traction is being applied gently upwards. Do not pull and pluck the ureter out. In such cases, where there is a lot of induration and one cannot develop the planes, try locating the ureter by feeling it and expose it by gentle sharp dissection.

Fig. 3.26f

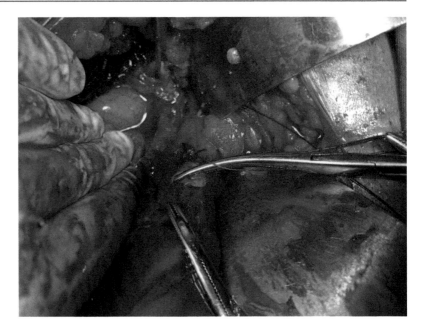

Take it on a tape wherever it has been exposed. Now, this will serve as a landmark, and the course of the ureter will be downward and medial toward the trigone of bladder. If one remains above this point throughout the dissection, then one can be assured that the ureter will not be injured.

The uterine artery has been cut, and the cut ends are held by clamps. The lumen of the artery is much smaller than the lumen of the ureter. But not always! Sometimes, ovarian artery can be very big, especially in cases of big adnexal masses. If one has any doubt *whether the tubular structure is the ureter, an artery, or a fallopian tube* (one can have this doubt if one cannot trace the tube to the fimbrial end because it is not visible due to adhesions), just feel it and stimulate it with a blunt instrument. Ureter will feel like a cord that slips between the fingers and will show peristalsis. After clamping and cutting, if the tubular structure shows blood coming out of the lumen, then it has to be a blood vessel! Just check the color of urine after cutting the structure. If the urine is clear, then probably the ureter is safe.

7. Figure 3.26g, the big arrow on the right side of the image points to the ureter taken on a tape, and the other two arrows show the cut ends of the uterine artery. The uterine arteries are above the level of the ureter, and the ureter takes a sharp medial turn at the level of the isthmus and the ischial spine to enter the tunnel of Wertheim. As one can see, the ureter is not visible/cannot be exposed throughout its course. There is a significant induration, and the planes are not well formed. The oozing can be appreciated. The fact that the clamps have been applied well above the point where the ureter has been exposed is reassuring because the ureter will only course downward toward the trigone of bladder.

Fig. 3.26g

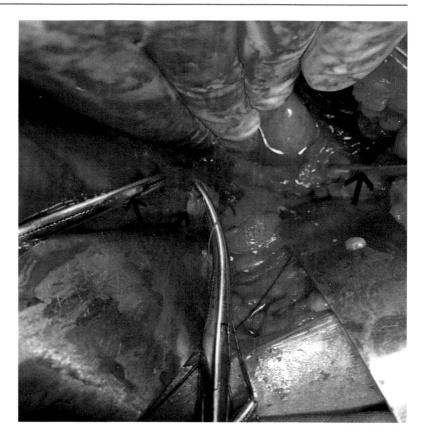

How to Locate the Ureter When There is no Identifiable Round Ligament (Figs. 3.27a–d, 3.28a–f)?

1. There is no round ligament identified (Fig. 3.27a). This is due to the fact that the patient has undergone hysterectomy previously. A fold of peritoneum on the lateral pelvic wall is held with artery forceps. Open it after making sure that there is nothing underneath.
2. Open the posterior peritoneum (Fig. 3.27b). Use sharp dissection, if necessary. Remember that do not force open and rip anything apart.

The structure being held by an Allis forceps (only the tip seen) is a fold of peritoneum, thickened because of adhesions from previous surgery.

3. Gently cut the peritoneum little by little (Fig. 3.27c). Feel with your fingers if there is anything underneath the peritoneal fold. Insert a thin Deaver's retractor and expose gently.

The ureter is now exposed. Gently stimulate it with a blunt instrument and look for peristalsis for confirmation. Take it on a tape if necessary. This will lateralize the ureter and will help in preventing injuries.

Fig. 3.27a

Fig. 3.27b

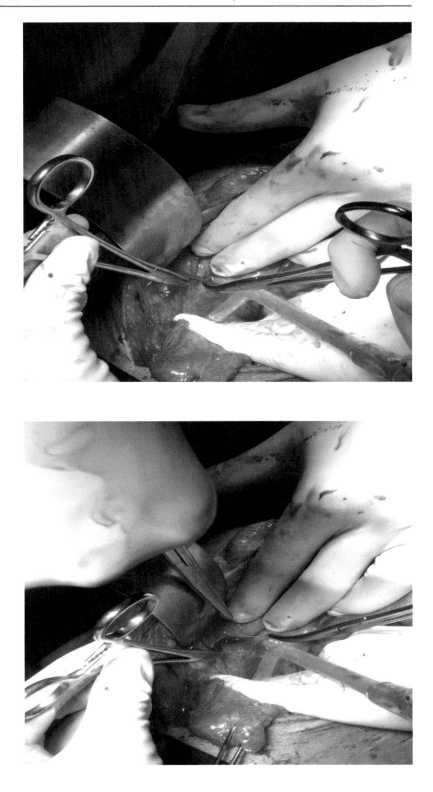

Fig. 3.27c

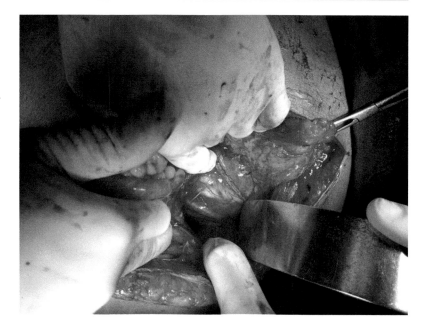

4. Panoramic view showing the exposed ureter (Fig. 3.27d). This patient has undergone two suboptimal surgeries, previously. The adnexa had been removed entirely leaving behind the uterus, and the patient continued to have persistent pain. One can see that a vertical incision has been taken. The first surgery was done laparoscopically and the second surgery was done through a transverse incision.

There is no round ligament identifiable to serve as a starting point. The ureter and the iliac vessels have been exposed by following the above technique—hold a fold of peritoneum in the lateral pelvic wall and slowly open it after making sure that there is no structure underneath.

A patient had undergone abdominal hysterectomy, following which she developed carcinoma ovary. She underwent neoadjuvant chemotherapy and has now been taken up for laparotomy for the removal of residual disease (Fig. 3.28a). As one can see, there is no ovary visible. In fact the pelvis is "empty" except for the rectum posteriorly and bladder anteriorly!

The fold of peritoneum along the lateral wall is being held (Fig. 3.28b). There is no structure underneath the fold.

Figure 3.28c shows another view of the same step. Here one can see transperitoneally that there is no structure seen under the fold of peritoneum.

The retroperitoneal space has been opened and the iliac vessels and the ureter is exposed (Fig. 3.28d). But where is the ovary?

Now the residual ovarian mass has become visible (Fig. 3.28e). The arrow is pointing toward it.

The residual ovarian mass can now be safely removed (Fig. 3.28f). One can appreciate that the ureter is located very close to it. Oozing is also apparent. But once the ureters have been localized and lateralized, one can excise the ovary and cauterize the bleeding vessels without fear of any injuries.

Fig. 3.27d

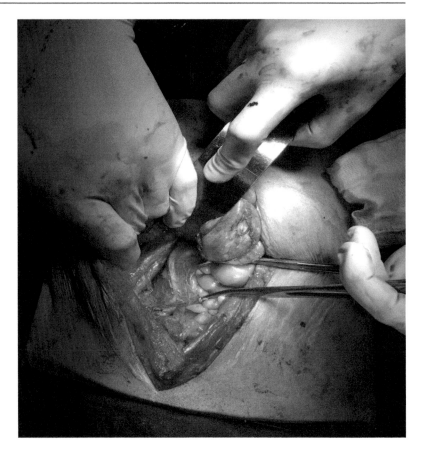

Fig. 3.28a

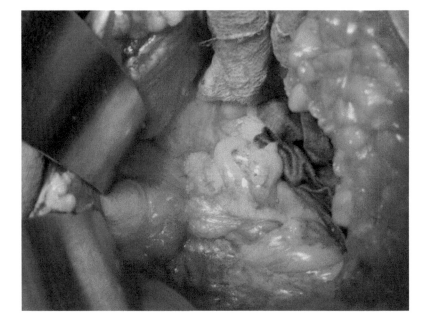

Fig. 3.28b

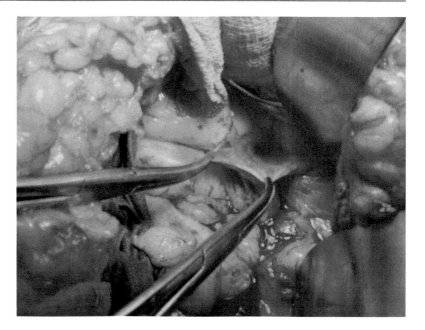

Fig. 3.28c

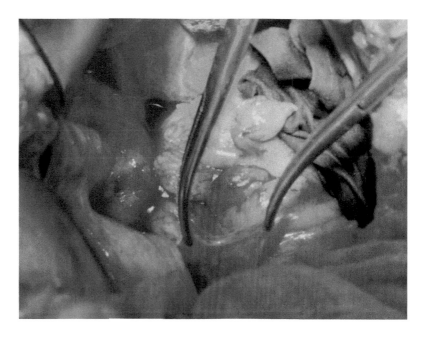

Fig. 3.28d

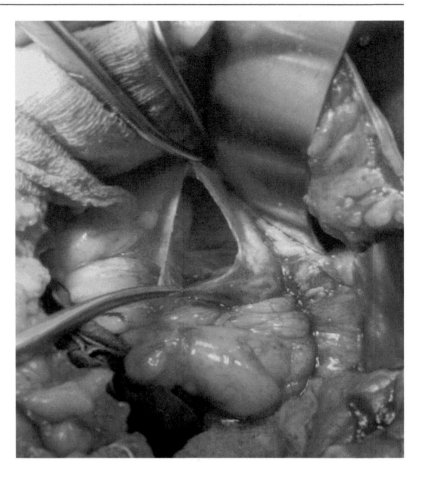

Fig. 3.28e

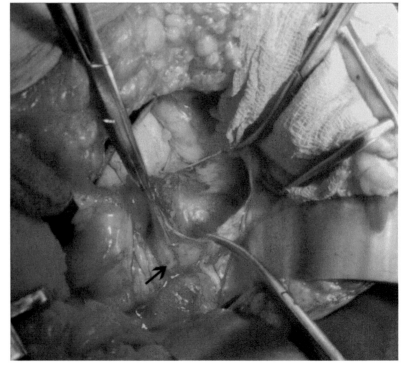

Fig. 3.28f

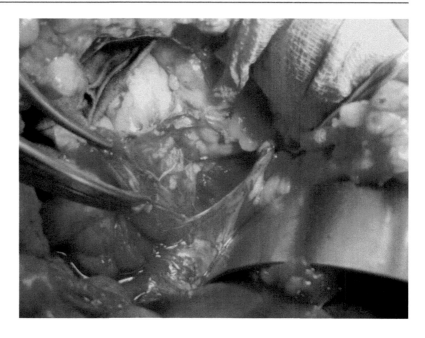

References

1. Mesdaghinia M, Abedzadeh-Kalaroudi M, Hedayati M, Moussavi-Bioki N. Iatrogenic gastrointestinal injuries during obstetrical and gynecological operation. Arch Trauma Res. 2013;2(2):81–4.
2. Moreira CM, Amaral E. Use of electrocautery for coagulation and wound complications in caesarean sections. Sci World J. 2014;2014:602375.
3. Siddaiah-Subramanya M, Tiang KW, Nyandowe M. Complications, implications, and prevention of electrosurgical injuries: corner stone of diathermy use for junior surgical trainees. Surg J (N Y). 2017;3(4):e148–53.
4. Engelsgjerd JS, LaGrange CA. Ureteral injury. StatPearls Publishing: Treasure Island; 2018.
5. Burks FN, Santucci RA. Management of iatrogenic ureteral injury. Ther Adv Urol. 2014;6(3):115–24.
6. Prowle JR, et al. Oliguria as predictive biomarker of acute kidney injury in critically ill patients. Crit Care. 2011;15(4):R172.
7. Duron J, et al. Adhesive postoperative small bowel obstruction: incidence and risk factors of recurrence after surgical treatment. Ann Surg. 2006;244(5):750–7.
8. Attard JP, Maclean AR. Adhesive small bowel obstruction: epidemiology, biology and prevention. Can J Surg. 2007;50(4):291–300.
9. Alpanes M, Gonzales-Casbas JM, Sanchez J, Pian H, Escobar-Morreale HF. Management of postmenopausal virilization. J Clin Endocrinol Metabol. 2012;97(8):2584–8.
10. El-Khalfaoui K, Bois A, Heitz, Kurzeder C, Sehouli J, Harter P. Current and future options in the management and treatment of uterine sarcoma. Ther Adv Med Oncol. 2014;6(1):21–8.

Part II

Special Situations

Frozen Pelvis: *How to Proceed?*

4

Frozen pelvis is a condition where dense adhesions due to any condition can result in pelvic structures becoming densely adhered and fixed to each other and to the pelvic walls. This could be due to endometriosis, pelvic inflammation (tuberculosis or otherwise), multiple previous surgeries, etc. [1, 2].

Note: The examples shown in Figs. 3.27a–d *and* 3.28a–f *are not that of frozen pelvis. The bowels and the pelvic structures are not plastered to each other or to the abdominopelvic walls. There is no significant adhesion formation; the problem in these situations is how to locate the ureter given the fact that there are no surgical landmarks.*

The general rules of operating in a frozen pelvis are

– Open the abdomen through a vertical incision or preferably first insert a laparoscope by the open method. There could be dense adhesions right under the umbilicus, and open method would be safer though not fool proof. Examine the peritoneal cavity and decide if the case can be accomplished laparoscopically or will laparotomy be necessary. If the abdomen has been opened by a transverse incision inadvertently, decide if the surgery can be accomplished by converting the incision to a Maylard incision. Otherwise, close the abdomen and explain to patient and relatives that the in situ findings were far more complicated than what

was determined by clinical evaluation and imaging. Plan a laparotomy through a vertical incision at a later date. This option is ideal if the disease is not an emergency condition. *Remember surgery is a diagnostic tool and one should not be embarrassed to have opened the abdomen just to find out what the disease is. Explain this confidently and patients will understand.*

The other option is to convert the incision into an inverted T incision. This is the least cosmetically preferred incision and is associated with higher postoperative morbidity and a higher risk of future incisional hernia (as compared to vertical incision). Trying to operate in the upper abdomen through a transverse incision can lead to suboptimal surgery, and the chances of visceral injuries are high.

To proceed with the dissection

– Use sharp dissection always. The dense adhesions would have plastered the bowels to each other and to the pelvic structures. The adherent bowels should not be separated by peeling or by blunt dissection with wet or dry gauze.
– Try and locate the round ligament and take a stay suture on it. Cut it and open the retroperitoneal space. Locate the ureter and take it on a tape if required. This will lateralize the ureter and keep it away from the operating field.

© Springer Nature Singapore Pte Ltd. 2020
A. R. Podder, J. G Seshadri, *Atlas of Difficult Gynecological Surgery*,
https://doi.org/10.1007/978-981-13-8173-7_4

- If one cannot locate the round ligament, catch a fold of peritoneum in the lateral wall of pelvis with a forceps. Open it after confirming that there is no vessel or tubular structure underneath. Gently extend the opening millimeter by millimeter and locate the ureter.
- If the patient has received previous radiation, let us say for carcinoma cervix, it will be difficult to reach the internal iliac artery. So remember that if one encounters profuse bleeding, it will be very difficult to do internal iliac artery ligation to control hemorrhage. Similarly, be cautious while separating the uterovesical fold. The chances of bladder injuries are high and so is the risk of developing vesicovaginal fistula.

Let us now study some photographs taken from a case where an in situ finding of frozen pelvis was found.

Frozen pelvis (Fig. 4.1a–g).

An example of frozen pelvis (Fig. 4.1a)—the loops of small intestine are adherent and fixed to one another and to the pelvic structures on account of dense adhesions. The appearance of the small intestines is also not normal. The rectus muscle has been divided to facilitate better exposure, and the upper cut end is held by a Babcock forceps.

Due to previous surgery, the muscles of the abdominal wall are densely adherent to the rectus sheath and the peritoneum below.

One has to remember that the bowel loops can get injured easily. Wrap the business end of the retractor with a wet mop if necessary to avoid trauma due to retraction. Ask for more assistants for retraction and increase the length of incision if necessary. The cosmetic problem of a large incision and future risk of incisional hernia are less important when compared to the possibility of injuring vital structures due to poor visualization and excessive retraction.

The pelvis-after the loops of intestine have been separated by sharp dissection and packed away (Fig. 4.1b). Nothing can be made out clearly as yet. What is the structure as indicated by the arrow pointing down? The arrow pointing up is showing a small white structure, is that the ovary? What is one supposed to remove when one encounters a case like this? So far, the bowel adhesions have been released, but what does one do from now? In a situation like this, the operating gynecologists might think *why did I open the abdomen? To remove what?* But if the preoperative imaging showed a uterus and adnexal structures, they must be there buried under the dense adhesions.

Fig. 4.1a

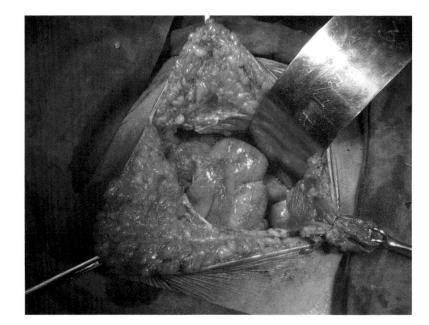

Fig. 4.1b

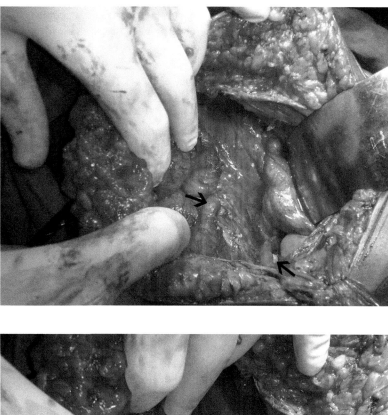

Fig. 4.1c

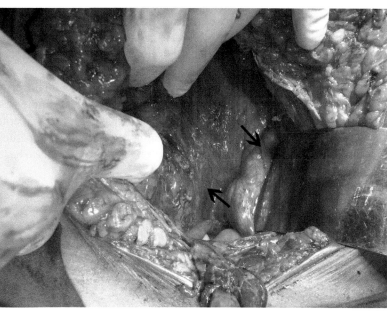

In Fig. 4.1c, the doubtful structure that was present in the previous image is not there. Instead we can see oozing in the posterior peritoneum. The arrow pointing up is showing an area of oozing, which looks like thin-walled friable vessels on the posterior peritoneum. The posterior peritoneum also appears to be plastered to the underlying structures, and it is not easy to lift a fold and open. There could be thin-walled friable veins below which can get easily traumatized and bleed profusely. The arrow pointing down is pointing to the mesosigmoid which has been retracted using Deaver's retractor.

The most important vital structure in the pelvis that is vulnerable to injury during gynecological surgeries is the ureter. One must first locate this organ; once it has been located (and correctly identified!), it is unlikely that the operating gynecologist will injure it.

As one can see (Fig. 4.1c), the dissection in the pelvis has begun and so has the oozing. One cannot clamp, cut, or ligate anything (that one is not sure of) before confirming the location of the ureter.

Now, the sharp dissection has made the fundus of the uterus obvious (Fig. 4.1d). It was buried deep under the adhesions. The fundus is being held by a Babcock forceps. The arrow is pointing to what looks like the fallopian tube; we can dissect along the structure to trace the fimbria. The ovary must be buried underneath. In this image, one can certainly appreciate that the peritoneum is plastered to the underlying structures. The round ligament is not standing out as a separate structure. The uterovesical fold is also densely adherent. Sharp dissection will be necessary. One has to be careful since bladder is vulnerable to injuries.

The right round ligament has been located and is held with an Allis forceps (Fig. 4.1e). The left round ligament is being held by a Babcock's forceps. The round ligament extends from the cornua to the lateral pelvic wall where it enters the inguinal canal. Now this can be clamped and cut. A stay suture on the lateral cut end of the round ligament will serve as a landmark for the rest of the surgery. Once the retroperitoneal space is

opened, one must slowly and carefully locate the ureter either by exposing it or should at least feel it—a cord that slips between the fingers.

The arrow is pointing to a nodular structure. This is just a fold of peritoneum. It is not the ovary, or the fallopian tube, and certainly not the ureter. The ureter is a retroperitoneal structure; it has to be exposed in order to be seen even in a clean case with no distortion of anatomy. However, one can sometimes see the ureter transperitoneally in the pouch of Douglas if there are no adhesions.

One can also see a thin-walled vessel above this nodular structure. The importance of not using any kind of force should be well appreciated.

Figure 4.1f is the close-up view of Fig. 4.1e. Now the retroperitoneal space is being entered by dividing the round ligament. One can appreciate that the peritoneum is plastered, and bleeding has started. One should proceed by hold the bleeding point by a fine tip forceps and cauterizing them, making sure it is just "touch and go." The cautery settings have to be checked before cauterization. And also one must take care not to force open any space with fingers or an instrument. The iliac veins will certainly be friable and due to the fact that the posterior peritoneum is plastered to the underlying retroperitoneal structures, one can expect the veins to be located very close— some-

Fig. 4.1d

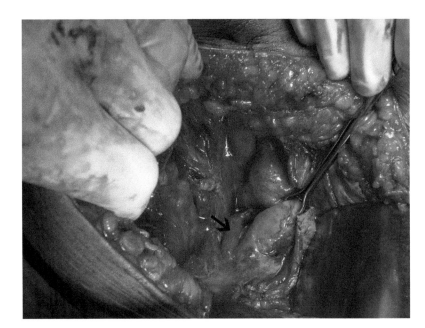

Fig. 4.1e

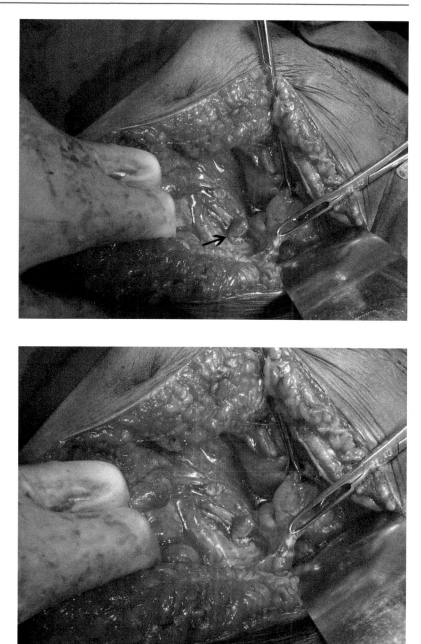

Fig. 4.1f

times just below and they might get traumatized and start bleeding profusely.

And now the ureter has been finally traced (Fig. 4.1g). It is the tubular structure in the retroperitoneal space as shown by the arrow. The cut end of the infundibulopelvic ligament is being held with a Babcock forceps; the atrophic ovary can be seen below the stump of the infundibulopelvic ligament. The rest of the sur-

gery should now not be very difficult, with the ureter having been located and can now be kept out of the operating field. The bladder position can be confirmed time to time by feeling the bulb of the Foley catheter. As stated earlier, and also evident in the previous images, the uterovesical fold is densely adherent, and separating the bladder will have to be done carefully, and by sharp dissection.

Fig. 4.1g

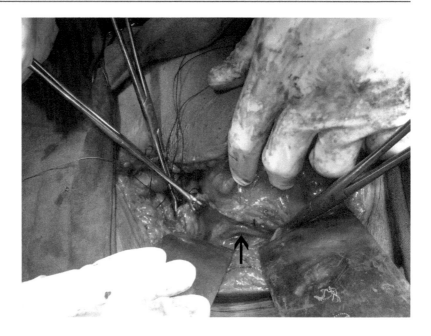

References

1. Mohling SI, Elkattah R, Furr RS. Endometriosis: tools for the frozen pelvis. J Minim Invasive Gynecol. 2015;22(6):S139.

2. De La Hera-Lazara, et al. Radical surgery for endometriosis: analysis of quality of life and surgical procedure. Clin Med Insights Womens Health. 2016;9:7–11.

Ovarian Tumor: *Challenges During Surgery*

5

This section is written with a general/laparoscopic gynecologist in mind, most of whom would not want to operate on malignancies, but come across malignant ovarian tumors occasionally and unexpectedly, usually as a case of an adnexal mass or a suspected leiomyoma which turns out to be malignant. Ovarian tumors with ascites and/or pleural effusion, omental cake, and very high CA-125 levels are always malignant (unless, it is a rare case of Meig's syndrome where there is pleural effusion, ascites, and it is due to a benign ovarian fibroma [1]), and such instances are usually not associated with unexpected findings on the operating table. Benign conditions with extensive adhesions or those cases where a benign appearing tumor turns out to be malignant on table are the situations which can be a challenge for a gynecologist.

A skilled surgeon may be capable of operating on a complicated case very easily and confidently, but to get the best results during surgery, every surgeon, whether skilled or a beginner, must keep in mind a few points during the preoperative evaluation of the patient. A few "simple" mistakes can ruin the best of intentions.

One of the commonest on table surprises a gynecologist can have is a leiomyoma (suspected and confirmed on imaging) turning out to be an ovarian tumor. The possibility of an ovarian tumor being malignant or borderline should be kept in mind till the definitive histopathology report becomes available even if other features are suggestive of a benign tumor. Borderline tumors are a separate entity with a unique behavior of their own, they can recur after removal, and can uncommonly undergo malignant transformation [2]. Even small ovarian tumors with no sold cystic areas, or ascites, can turn out to be malignant. Tumor marker levels can be normal preoperatively in a good number of malignant ovarian tumors. Frozen section should be kept ready before operating on every case of ovarian tumor, though even in the best of centers the correlation between frozen section and final histopathology is not 100% [3]. If the presence of an ovarian tumor is a surprise finding (e.g., if the preoperative diagnosis was leiomyoma), then one can go ahead with the procedure even if there is no frozen section available. But inform the patient (once she is out of anesthesia and is feeling better) and relatives that restaging might be necessary should the final histopathology report show malignancy or a borderline tumor. This can be the case even when frozen section is available, since there can be a discrepancy between frozen section and the final histopathology reports.

If there are features of malignancy on table, or if consent for loss of fertility has not been taken, close the abdomen and plan a staging procedure at a later date. *Remember that surgery is a diagnostic tool, and one should not be embarrassed to have opened the abdomen just to find out what the disease is. Explain this confidently and patients will understand.*

© Springer Nature Singapore Pte Ltd. 2020
A. R. Podder, J. G Seshadri, *Atlas of Difficult Gynecological Surgery*,
https://doi.org/10.1007/978-981-13-8173-7_5

For this reason, whenever an ovarian/adnexal mass is encountered by a gynecologist in outpatient consultation, a per rectal examination to assess the nodularity and fixity is a must. Upper GI endoscopy to rule out any possibility of GI malignancy and the ovarian mass being a metastatic tumor should be considered if clinical features are suggestive. Krukenberg tumors of the ovary are rare [4]. They are metastatic ovarian tumors with stomach carcinoma, colorectal carcinoma, breast carcinoma, being the commonest primary malignancies. Metastatic tumors of the ovary can also be due to hematogenous malignancies. They are usually bilateral with the ovaries being moderately enlarged with an irregular surface and generally free of adhesions. Ascites is present in nearly half of the cases. CA-125 levels are raised though not very grossly. Thus they can be mistaken to be a simple case of an ovarian tumor. Though ovarian metastasectomy may have a role in certain cases, Krukenberg tumors have a poor prognosis [4, 5]. Therefore, it would be wise to do a thorough preoperative assessment and not be in a hurry to operate. It is important to do a breast examination as a part of routine gynecological examination since breast lesions are common and can actually be the primary in the rare event of the ovarian tumor being a metastatic tumor. Also, peripheral smear is important and should be done as a part of CBC. The ovarian tumor can be a metastatic tumor due to a primary hematogenous malignancy.

A normal CA-125 can be a feature of early malignancy before the tumor has spread in a good number of patients [6]. Germ cell tumors are more likely in young girls and ideally all tumor markers-CA-125, alpha-fetoprotein, LDH, and beta hCG, should be done in all patients with an adnexal mass [7]. If a granulosa cell tumor is suspected, then an endometrial biopsy to rule out endometrial hyperplasia and carcinoma endometrium due to hyperestrogenic state should be done preoperatively [8, 9]. And if the granulosa cell tumor is detected for the first time on table by frozen section, then one should be prepared to expect endometrial hyperplasia or carcinoma endometrium also to be present. If the patient has completed her family and if the surgery planned includes hysterectomy, then one must immediately proceed to do the staging and completion of surgery. Granulosa cell tumors of the ovary

are low-grade malignancies with a slow indolent growth and are known to secrete estrogen [8]. Carcinoma endometrium which can arise due to unopposed estrogen can be more aggressive than the granulosa cell tumor itself. If the patient is young and desires fertility, or if the consent has not been recorded before the start of the surgery, then one must close the abdomen and inform the patient about the need for repeat surgery for staging and completion of surgery. Fertility conserving options can be explored depending on the stage and grade.

If granulosa cell tumor is detected for the first time after the final histopathology report is ready, then again, the patient should be counseled about the need for staging and completion of surgery.

In fact, during preoperative evaluation, one must suspect the possibility of endometrial hyperplasia and carcinoma endometrium if there is a history of irregular and excessive or postmenopausal bleeding, or if there is an associated hyperestrogenic state like PCOD or anovulatory cycles. The imaging report should be carefully studied. Apart from noting findings like enlarged lymph nodes, loss of fat planes, etc., one must look for ET, and if this is significant for patient's age, then a preoperative endometrial biopsy is indicated. Patients taking tamoxifen should also be counseled to report any vaginal bleeding promptly to rule out the possibility of endometrial hyperplasia and carcinoma endometrium [10].

The ovarian tumor (or whatever the gynecological condition which has been detected preoperatively) could be benign, but there could be complex atypical endometrial hyperplasia or carcinoma endometrium, which has been missed in the preoperative assessment.

All these measures will greatly help the gynecologist to avoid an intraoperative disaster. Remember that many times a fertility sparing surgery is what is being planned.

If the patient is a clear case of ovarian malignancy, then refer to or call a gynecologic/surgical oncologist to scrub in for surgery. Fertility-sparing surgeries in a patient with malignancy require a greater amount of documentation. It is better to close the abdomen after careful explanation to relatives than proceed with what might be a confused and a suboptimal surgery, with the patient herself not being involved in the decision-making.

Aspiration or FNAC is strongly discouraged since it will only upstage the tumor. It can however be done in a clear case of advanced ovarian tumor for the purpose of tissue diagnosis for neoadjuvant therapy [11].

But while operating a case of ovarian tumor, following points have to be kept in mind.

- Do the staging. Collect free fluid for cytology to rule out malignant cells. Flush the pouch of Douglas, the two paracolic gutters, and the two subdiaphragmatic spaces with saline and aspirate it for cytology. Take generous peritoneal biopsies and biopsies from any suspicious area or adhesions. This has to be done even if the tumor is certain to be benign. This can be done laparoscopically as well. If one is unable to remove all the visible evidence of the tumor, the residual disease can be removed by a repeat surgery at a later date (after neoadjuvant chemotherapy in cases of malignant ovarian tumor, or if the patient becomes symptomatic or has an increase in growth of the residual disease as in cases of endometriosis, leiomyoma, PID, etc.), but remember staging is something that is done only during the first surgery. So if staging is not done or done inadequately, then subsequent treatment will always be suboptimal if the tumor turns out to be malignant.
- Do not cause rupture of an intact and well-circumscribed tumor. It might lead to upstaging should the tumor be malignant.
- In case of ovarian torsion, it was earlier believed that once an ovarian tumor undergoes torsion, the blood supply and venous return get cut off. There will be anaerobic metabolism in cells and accumulation of lactic acid and toxic metabolites. Untwisting will release this into circulation. The more congested and purplish the tumor looks, more likely it is for it to contain toxic metabolites. However, recent studies suggest that detorsion can be safely done if ovarian function is desired. It can be done even if the twisted ovary looks swollen and congested [12]. However, if there is a tumor which needs to be removed, then there is no point in untwisting it. It should be removed intact and sent for frozen section.

Divide the round ligament, open the folds of broad ligament, locate the ureter, and then clamp, cut, and ligate the infundibulopelvic ligament. Ovarian tumors are particularly known for their proximity to the ureter, and one should not underestimate the importance of this step [13]. Remove the specimen and send it for frozen section, if available. And then proceed with the surgery (hysterectomy, if the patient is elderly/postmenopausal). If the frozen section report and the cytology report are positive for malignancy, then proceed with completion of surgery. If frozen section facility is not available, then it will take a week for the staging report and the definitive histopathology reports to arrive. Inform the patient and relatives, should the definitive histopathology show malignancy; then restaging with completion of surgery will be required.

Now let us study some photographs taken during surgery for ovarian tumor. In some cases, it was certain that the patient has a malignant ovarian tumor. In some other cases, it was a complete surprise on table. Sometimes even the presence of ovarian torsion can turn out to be a complete surprise.

Malignant Ovarian Tumor: A Surprise Finding (Fig. 5.1)

A picture of a huge ovarian tumor (Fig. 5.1); it looks malignant. There is no ascites, but presence of solid cystic areas is evident. The opposite ovary is also not entirely normal. However, there are no adhesions, and the uterus is normal. One cannot do a staging procedure with an incision of this size. Extend the incision; the under surface of the diaphragm, liver, the greater omentum will all have to be examined for deposits, for which a bigger incision will be needed.

Ovarian Tumors Can Be Huge! (Fig. 5.2a, b)

A large ovarian tumor which has been exteriorized, but the incision will have to be extended for a complete staging procedure (Fig. 5.2a). Do not hesitate to take a large incision; a suboptimal surgery through an inadequate incision with resulting injuries due to rough retraction and inadequate

Fig. 5.1

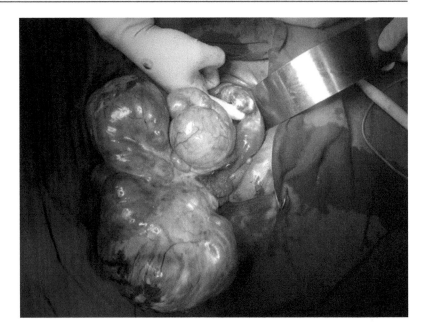

Fig. 5.2a

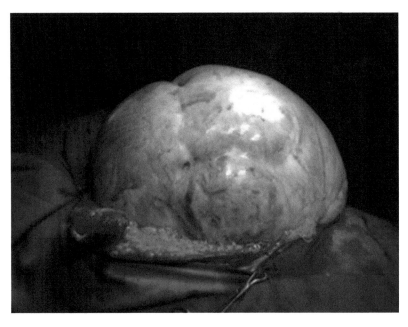

exposure are bigger problems than burst abdomen, cosmetic issues, and incisional hernia.

Burst abdomen is a serious complication with an incidence less than 5% in most centers [14]. It can occur even with small vertical and transverse incisions. It is associated with raised intraabdominal pressures in the postoperative period and wound infection. The predisposing factors which cause postoperative increase in intraabdominal pressure and wound infection need to be controlled in order to prevent burst abdomen.

The same ovarian tumor has been completely exteriorized without intraoperative spillage (Fig. 5.2b). Call for another assistant who can hold such a large and a heavy tumor. The tumor may be large, but it could well be benign or early stage malignancy. Mucinous tumors are known to attain large sizes. Rupture with intraoperative spillage will upstage tumors of stage IA and IB to IC. This could be a very big setback for young patients who have a long life and career ahead of them. So the importance of this precaution cannot be underestimated.

Fig. 5.2b

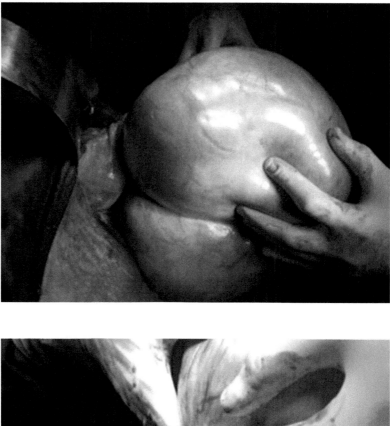

Fig. 5.3

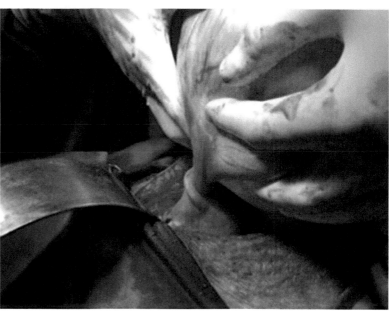

There Is a Torsion—One and Half Loops (Fig. 5.3)

Do not untwist it (Fig. 5.3); it is a large ovarian tumor which needs to be removed anyway; the patient is a middle-aged woman. Locate the ureter and then clamp, cut, and ligate the infundibulopelvic ligament after making sure that the ureter is away.

However, if it is a case of ovarian torsion in a young woman, then detorsion with cystectomy can be considered. Tissue viability and duration of torsion are important in deciding how much of the ovarian tissue should be sacrificed [12].

How to Avoid Injuring the Ureter While Clamping the Infundibulopelvic Ligament and How to Remove the Ovarian Tumor Intact Without Intra-operative Spillage
(Fig. 5.4a–e)

Check if there is something holding the tumor back (Fig. 5.4a). Any adhesions? Is it adhered to the bowel behind? Release the adhesions before pulling the tumor out, lest the tumor ruptures and result in intraoperative spillage.

Do not rush to clamp the infundibulopelvic ligament (Fig. 5.4b). The ureter may lie very close to it. First, divide the round ligament and confirm the location of the ureter. The assistant is holding the tumor, making sure that it does not wobble and obstruct the surgeon's view (Fig. 5.4b).

The ureter has been located as shown by the arrow (Fig. 5.4c). The infundibulopelvic ligament is being held by a Babcock forceps. Now, the infundibulopelvic ligament can be safely clamped, cut, and ligated. The tumor should be immediately sent for frozen section.

Fig. 5.4a

Fig. 5.4b

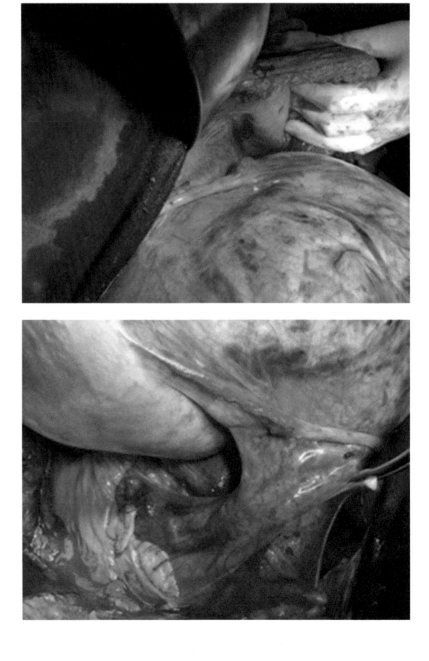

The infundibulopelvic ligament being clamped and divided; from a distance it looks so simple, but one has to remember that clamping the infundibulopelvic ligament is probably the most common site where the ureters can be injured [13] (Fig. 5.4d).

The entire tumor has been removed without rupture (Fig. 5.4e). A measuring scale has not been placed to indicate the size, but the tumor diameter is roughly as long as two curved clamps.

Fig. 5.4c

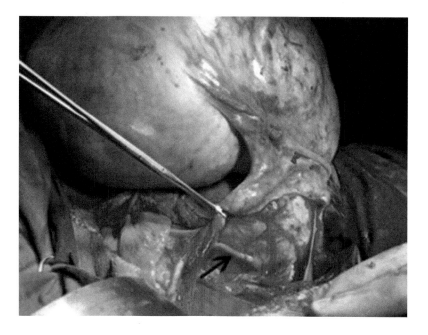

Fig. 5.4d

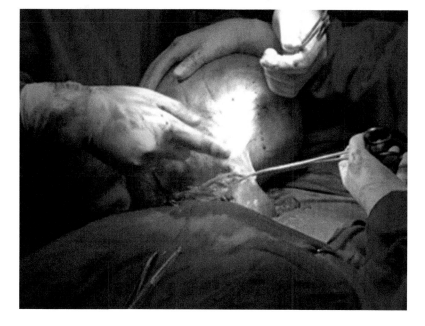

Fig. 5.4e

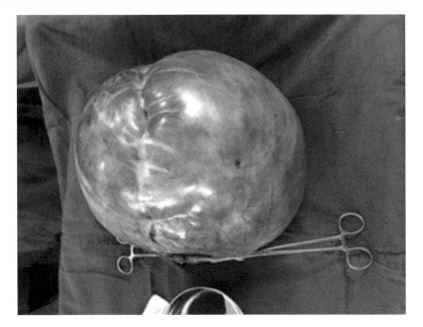

Fig. 5.5

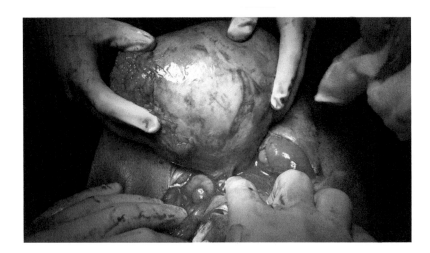

Ovarian Malignancy with Adhesions
(Figs. 5.5, 5.6a, b, 5.7, 5.8a, b, and 5.9a–d)

Figure 5.5 Shows an ovarian tumor which is adherent to the adjacent structures. The omentum has been divided, with a part of it still stuck to the tumor.

Collect free fluid for cytology. Examine the entire peritoneal cavity; take samples of any suspicious looking nodules and adhesions. Take large peritoneal biopsies. If the frozen section suggests malignancy, proceed to do

the complete surgery with pelvic and para-aortic lymphadenectomy and total omentectomy. Call for help and extra assistants. In an obese woman, one will require two assistants just for retracting the obese abdomen. Do not approach the para-aortic space through a small incision.

Such a case should not be attempted in the first place without keeping assistants and frozen section ready. If one is not prepared to do a complete surgery and if a gynecologic-oncologist/oncosurgeon cannot be called to scrub in, then remove the tumor, do a thorough staging, and

Fig. 5.6a

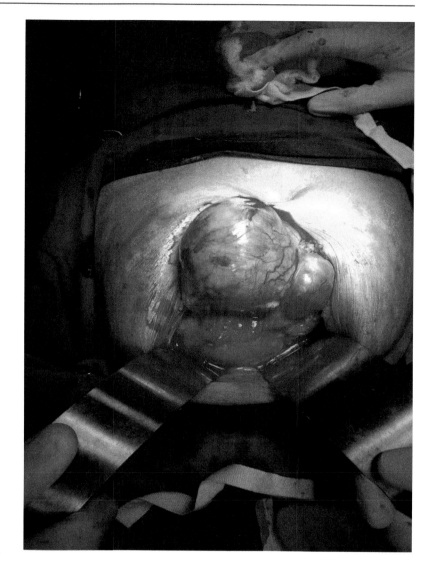

Fig. 5.6b

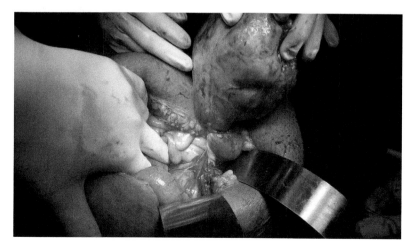

Fig. 5.7

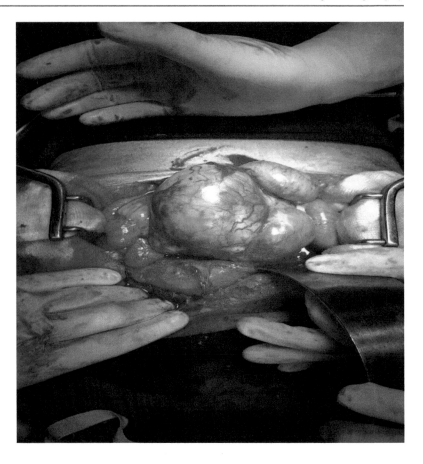

Fig. 5.8a

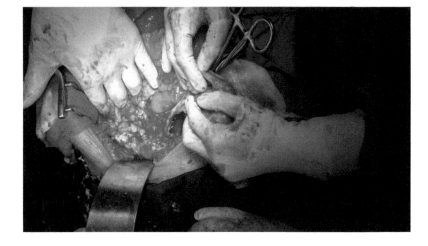

close. Refer the patient to the appropriate surgeon or reschedule the case with a gynecologic-
oncologist/oncosurgeon at a later date (but this
may not be possible if an injury to the bowel
while opening the abdomen has occurred or if
torrential bleeding has started). But do not skip
the staging, this cannot be done later. Completion
of surgery can be done later, but not staging! A
very important point, gynecologists have to keep
in mind always.

Fig. 5.8b

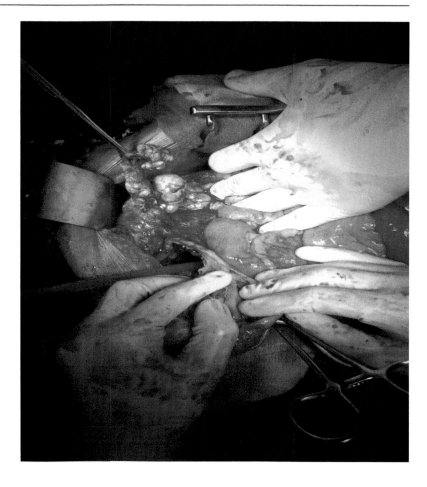

Fig. 5.9a

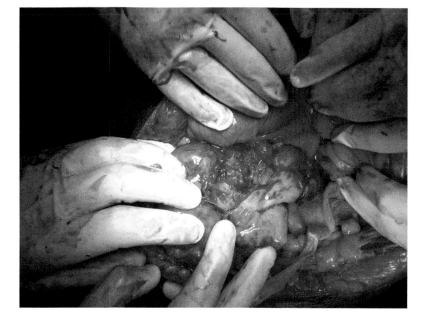

Fig. 5.9b

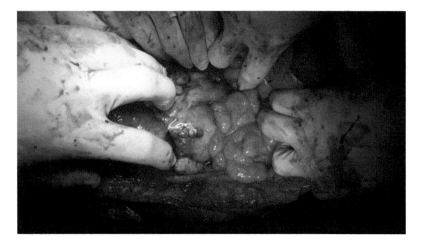

Fig. 5.9c

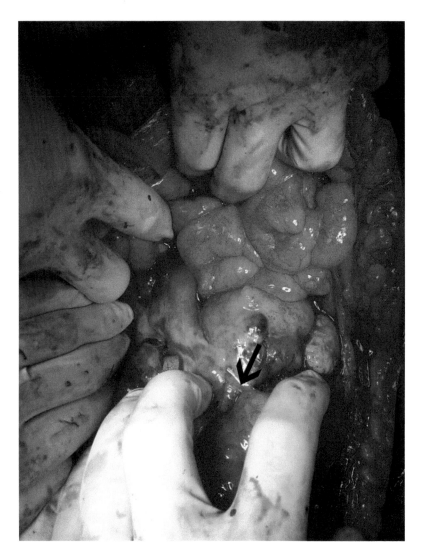

Fig. 5.9d

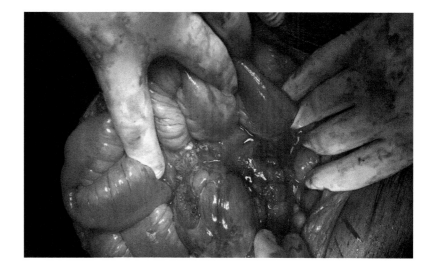

Fertility sparing surgery for borderline ovarian tumors and well-differentiated, early stage ovarian malignancy (stage IA) is possible [15, 16]. Apart from extensive documentation, the gynecologist has to impress upon the patient that she must come regular follow-ups for early diagnosis of recurrence and for completion of surgery once child bearing is complete. Fertility-sparing surgery in minor girls with well-differentiated early stage malignancy requires ethical clearances [17].

The incision is grossly inadequate, extend it further (Fig. 5.6a). At the lower end, it is obvious that the tumor is stuck to the fundus of the uterus. Deposits on the serosa of the uterus are also evident. It is clear that it is a malignant ovarian tumor. A complete staging is a must.

Now the incision has been extended well above the umbilicus (Fig. 5.6b). Adhesions between the posterior surface of the uterus and bowel are now seen. The tumor can now be removed. There is no rupture or intraoperative spillage. The staging will now be done. The specimen will be sent to lab for frozen section, and the report can be expected by the time the staging and hysterectomy (the patient has completed her family and does not want to conserve her uterus) are complete. Lymphadenectomy and total omentectomy will follow once the frozen section report confirms malignancy.

Another example of an ovarian tumor adherent to the fundus of the uterus (Fig. 5.7)—the incision needs to be extended further.

The tumor has unfortunately ruptured causing intraoperative spillage (Fig. 5.8a). But there are deposits everywhere in the pelvis and beyond. It is pretty certain that it is a case of carcinoma ovary stage IIIC; the malignancy has spread beyond the pelvis with deposits >2 cm. So the question of upstaging due to intraoperative spillage does not arise in this case.

Proceeding with completion of surgery (Fig. 5.8b)-all the nodules, metastatic deposits, and suspicious looking adhesions have to be excised. The suction cannula is suctioning out the contents of the ruptured ovarian tumor. The adhesion between the posterior surface of the uterus and bowel will have to be separated by sharp dissection.

If complete debulking is not possible, then one has the option of doing a thorough staging and closing the abdomen. The patient can be referred for neoadjuvant chemotherapy and assessed for the removal of residual disease after three cycles of chemotherapy. After the completion of surgery, the patient will have to take adjuvant chemotherapy.

Another example of what is certainly a case of carcinoma ovary (Fig. 5.9a). It is obvious that the case is stage III- the disease has spread beyond the pelvis.

Now, this can be an expected or an unexpected finding. The patient's age, symptoms, grossly raised preoperative CA-125 levels, and imaging reports may be virtually confirmatory of ovarian malignancy. But there are many benign conditions where CA-125 can be significantly raised. The patient may be young, and the imaging report may show a moderate-sized ovarian tumor with no ascites. There could be extensive deposits in pouch of Douglas in patients with endometriosis. On the contrary, a patient with a clinical picture of leiomyoma could turn out to be a case of ovarian malignancy. So how can one decide if the condition is benign or malignant preoperatively? One cannot possibly prepare every patient with an adnexal mass for surgery as a potentially malignant case since most adnexal masses are benign. Per rectal examination preoperatively can be very informative. Hard fixed nodular deposits and involvement of the rectovaginal fascia is strongly suggestive of malignancy.

Should one find advanced ovarian malignancy on table when the preoperative diagnosis was that of a benign condition, then one must do a complete staging. If the case has started laparoscopically, then one can do a staging laparoscopy or take a vertical incision and proceed with a staging laparotomy. If one is not prepared to do a complete surgery, then one can close the abdomen after staging. It is better to do a thorough staging and close and then refer or reschedule the case with proper consent and counseling, rather than proceeding to do an incomplete staging and removal.

Now it is obvious that the ovarian tumor is malignant (Fig. 5.9b), so therefore proceeding with staging and completion of surgery. But the first step would be to look for planes from where one can begin dissection.

The arrow is pointing at the junction where dissection can begin (Fig. 5.9c). The ovarian tumor, fundus of the uterus, and the small intestine are all fused at this point.

The dissection has begun, and one can expect a lot of bleeding (Fig. 5.9d). Tumor is densely adherent to the rectum and sigmoid.

The options for a gynecologist are

– If it is not possible to proceed with the surgery in a small setup, then take biopsies and close. Do not extend the incision if the intention is not to do staging and/or completion of the surgery. There is no question of upstaging the tumor by taking biopsies when deposits are seen all over the abdomen. It has to be minimum stage IIIC. But taking biopsies or causing intraoperative spillage in what could be an early stage tumor is a very gross mistake. Similarly doing FNAC preoperatively is also discouraged since it will upstage an early disease. But if there is an extensive disease, then taking FNAC from the tumor, or the omental cake, or ascitic or pleural tap for histological evidence to start neoadjuvant chemotherapy is justified, since the question of upstaging does not arise [18, 19]. The presence of hepatic metastasis (stage IV), malignant pleural effusion (stage IV), omental cake (stage IIIC), and large peritoneal deposits >2 cm (stage IIIC) are all suggestive of advanced disease. So obviously, the question of further upstaging does not arise.

One can refer the patient to a gynecologic oncologist/oncosurgeon or for neoadjuvant chemotherapy. But the question arises—was the preoperative evaluation done thoroughly? The extensive deposits should have been detected in preoperative imaging.

If an experienced surgeon can be called to scrub in, then one can go ahead with staging and completion of surgery.

Locating the Ureter in a Case of Advanced Ovarian Malignancy (Fig. 5.10a–c)

How to locate the ureter in such situation—advanced malignancy with extensive tumor deposits (Fig. 5.10a). First, take a fold of peritoneum laterally in the pelvis.

Now check if there is any structure felt underneath the fold with fingers (Fig. 5.10b). When it is certain that there is nothing beneath, make a small nick and open the retroperitoneal space. Slowly and carefully extend the opening and

Fig. 5.10a

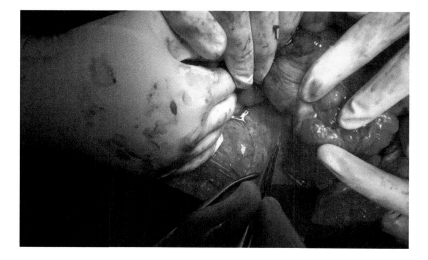

Fig. 5.10b

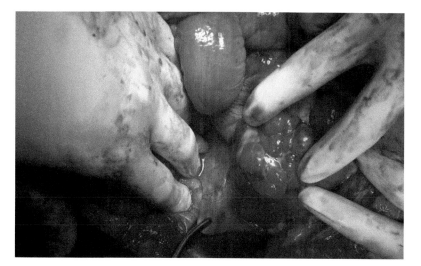

Fig. 5.10c

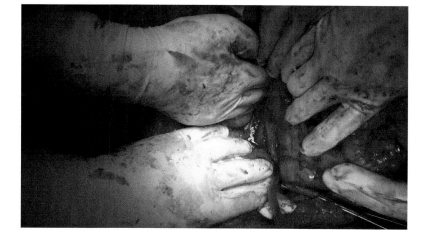

locate the ureter. One can feel for a "cord that slips between fingers." Remember to use sharp dissection and not to force open a space if the planes are not well made out.

The ureter has been located (Fig. 5.10c). One can take it on a tape if there are lots of deposits in the pouch of Douglas. This will help lateralizing the ureter and one can remove all the deposits which are there in the pouch of Douglas.

In Fig. 5.10c, the infundibulopelvic ligament has been clamped and cut. The cut ovarian vessels can be appreciated in the pedicle which is being held in the clamp. One can apply a free tie and ligate the vessels and proceed with the dissection.

References

1. Saha S, Robertson M. Meigs' and pseudo-Meigs' syndrome. Australas J Ultrasound Med. 2012;15(1): 29–31.
2. Hauptmann S, Friedrich K, Redline R, Avril S. Ovarian borderline tumors in the 2014 WHO classification: evolving concepts and diagnostic criteria. Virchows Arch. 2017;470(2):125–42.
3. Hatami H, Mohsenifar Z, Alavi SN. The diagnostic accuracy of frozen section compared to permanent section: a single center study in Iran. Iran J Pathol. 2015;10(4):295–9.
4. Al-Agha OM, Nicastri AD. An in-depth look at Krukenberg tumor: an overview. Arch Pathol Lab Med. 2006;130(11):1725–30.
5. Wu F, et al. Clinical characteristics and prognostic analysis of Krukenberg tumor. Mol Clin Oncol. 2015;3(6):1323–8.
6. Menczer J, Ben-Shem E, Golan A, Levy T. The significance of normal pretreatment levels of CA125 (<35 U/mL) in epithelial ovarian carcinoma. Rambam Maimonides Med J. 2015;6(1):e0005.
7. Malati T, Kumari RG, Yadagiri B. Application of tumor markers in ovarian malignancies. Indian J Clin Biochem. 2001;16(2):224–33.
8. Bacalbasa N, Stoica C, Mirea G, Belescu I. Endometrial carcinoma associated with ovarian granulosa cell tumors—a case report. Anticancer Res. 2015;35(10):5547–50.
9. Ayhan A, Salman MC, Velipasaoglu M, Sakinci M, Yuce K. Prognostic factors in adult granulosa cell tumors of the ovary: a retrospective analysis of 80 cases. J Gynecol Oncol. 2009;20(3):158–63.
10. Korkmazer E, Solak N, Tokgoz VY. Assessment of thickened endometrium in tamoxifen therapy. Turk J Obstet Gynecol. 2014;11(4):215–8.
11. Ramljak V, Muhaxhiri MA, Kelcec IV. Cytology in diagnosis of ovarian cancer. Libri Oncol. 2015;43(1–3):33–9.
12. Huang C, Hong M, Ding D. A review of ovary torsion. Ci Ji Yi Xue Za Zhi. 2017;29(3):143–7.
13. Burks FN, Santucci RA. Management of iatrogenic ureteral injury. Ther Adv Urol. 2014;6(3):115–24.
14. van Ramshorst GH, et al. Abdominal wound dehiscence in adults: development and validation of a risk model. World J Surg. 2010;34(1):20–7.
15. Rema P, Ahmed I. Fertility sparing surgery in gynecologic cancer. J Obstet Gynaecol India. 2014;64(4):234–8.
16. Fiechtinger M, Rodriguez-Wallberg KA. Fertility preservation in women with cervical, endometrial or ovarian cancers. Gynecol Oncol Res Pract. 2016;3:8.
17. Bouchard-Fortier G, Kim RH, Allen L, Gupta A, May T. Fertility-sparing surgery for the management of young women with embryonal rhabdomyosarcoma of the cervix: a case series. Gynecol Oncol Rep. 2016;18:4–7.
18. Bandyopadhyay A, Chakraborty J, Chowdhury AR, Bhattacharya A, Bhattachrya P, Chowdhury MK. Fine needle aspiration cytology of ovarian tumors with histological correlation. J Cytol. 2012;29(1):35–40.
19. Mathur SR. Ovarian cancer: role of cytology. Indian J Med Paediatr Oncol. 2007;27(Suppl 1).

Densely Adherent Bladder: Dissection Technique

6

Densely adherent bladder can be found in cases of previous caesarean section [1, 2] and in those patients with the history of having undergone cervicopexy. One often encounters an advanced bladder while doing an LSCS in a patient of previous caesarean delivery(s). But if the lower segment is well formed at the time of repeat caesarean, it is usually not a problem opening the uterovesical fold and pushing the bladder down. The tissue edema actually helps the obstetrician get the right plane. The problem of separating the bladder is usually encountered when performing hysterectomy in cases of previous LSCS, endometriosis, PID, and malignancy.

In such situations, always use sharp dissection (the golden rule!) and stay close to the specimen. Feel the bulb of Foley catheter time to time and use it as a landmark. Hold a small bit of tissue with a blunt forceps, cauterize, and then cut the charred band using tissue cutting scissors. Try to go in this way as below as possible. Forcibly pushing the bladder down with a "peanut" or with a sponge on holder is strongly discouraged; it can traumatize the bladder and also cause profuse bleeding. One must remember that descending branch of the uterine artery, which supplies the cervix and vagina, can get traumatized leading to profuse hemorrhage. The vesical venous plexus can also get traumatized and bleeding from these vessels is very difficult to control. So the rule of the thumb is hold a small bit of tissue with fine tip forceps, cauterize, and cut close to the specimen.

If bleeding starts, put a mop and give gentle pressure and begin dissection from another point. If there is a lot of bleeding, maybe one is not in the correct plane. *Is the dissection going into the substance of the cervix?* Consider this possibility.

When using cautery near the base of bladder or near any vital structure, it is important to cauterize as "touch and go." This is because the tissue damage extends beyond the area of visible charring. The electrocautery settings have to be checked; it is advisable to keep it low. Should sparking occur or if dense charring of tissues noted, then immediately lower the electrocautery settings. Should profuse bleeding occur, then it may be advisable to do a bilateral internal iliac artery ligation than apply cautery or take deep stitches near the base of bladder. A mop can be placed on the bleeding area and the round ligaments divided (the round ligaments would have already been divided when one is opening the uterovesical fold, but if one wants to quickly access the internal iliac artery to ligate it to control pelvic hemorrhage, then one might have to divide the round ligaments again a bit laterally). The folds of the broad ligament should be separated, and the bifurcation of the common iliac artery located. The internal iliac artery is the medial branch of the common iliac artery.

Bladder injury can occur if precautions are not taken. Bladder can be injured as a result of excessive use of cautery or inadvertent stitches in the base of bladder. Injuries can also happen

© Springer Nature Singapore Pte Ltd. 2020
A. R. Podder, J. G Seshadri, *Atlas of Difficult Gynecological Surgery*,
https://doi.org/10.1007/978-981-13-8173-7_6

during sharp dissection, but in injuries due to sharp dissection, the edges are neat and clean and are easier to repair. And the injuries are almost always detected on table. But in case of injury due to excessive use of cautery or inadvertent stitches, the injury becomes evident after the devitalized tissues have sloughed away and a vesicovaginal or a ureterovaginal fistula has developed. The repair is complicated by the fact that the tissues are edematous and the edges are irregular.

If the base of bladder, trigone, or the ureter is involved, the repair requires a urologist. Rent in the base of bladder is not as simple as a rent in the dome of bladder. Ureteric orifices can get included during closure, further complicating the situation.

One may encounter a situation where one cannot clearly make out the cervicovaginal junction anteriorly. In such situations, try the posterior technique. Skeletonize the uterine arteries and ligate them. Now divide the uterosacral ligaments which are attached to the cervix at 5 o'clock and 7 o'clock positions separately, not including the Mackenrodt's ligaments. Open the fold of peritoneum below the cervix posteriorly, and open the vagina posteriorly. Hold the cervix with an Allis forceps and deliver the cervix into the pelvis. Ask the assistant to give upward traction to the specimen. Gently do sharp dissection and free the cervix from the vaginal attachments all around. Close the vagina making sure the bladder is not included in the vault sutures. If bladder injury is suspected, check the color of urine. Do retrograde filling of bladder with saline stained with methylene blue and see if any part of the bladder is included in the vault sutures. If methylene blue stained saline is seen pouring into the pelvis, then it is certain that there is a bladder rent.

Now let us study a series of photographs which illustrate how one must proceed with the dissection in a case of densely adherent bladder.

Fig. 6.1a

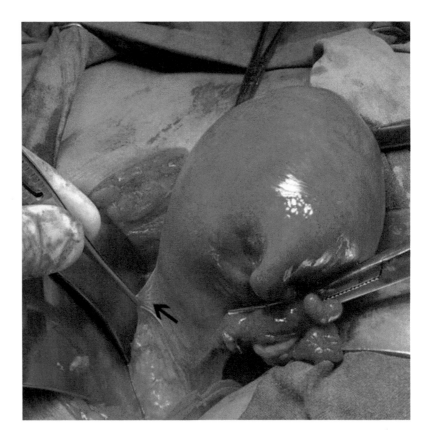

Sharp Dissection to Push the Bladder Down (Fig. 6.1a–i)

The dissection begins by holding the uterovesical fold with a forceps and cauterizing it (Fig. 6.1a). There could be vessels underneath, and incising the fold can lead to bleeding which can obscure the operating field. In the above case, the bladder is quite below. Locating the inflated bulb of Foleys catheter will confirm the position of the bladder.

The uterovesical fold has been opened and the dissection has begun (Fig. 6.1b), and it is clear that bleeding can be expected. Hold a small fold of tissue with a forceps and cauterize it. And then cut the cauterized tissue. Proceed little by little.

Remain close to the specimen throughout the procedure (Fig. 6.1c).

Fig. 6.1b

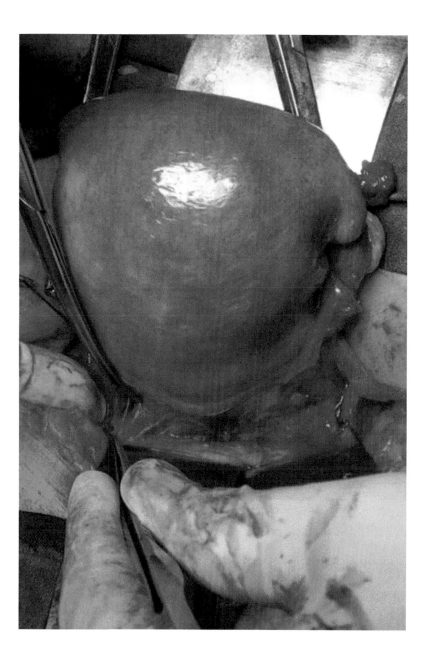

Fig. 6.1c

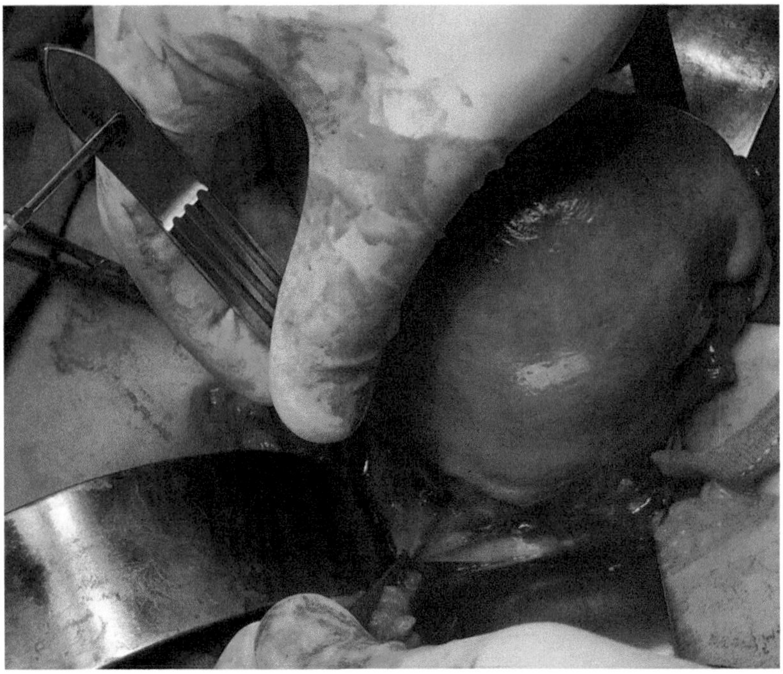

Fig. 6.1d

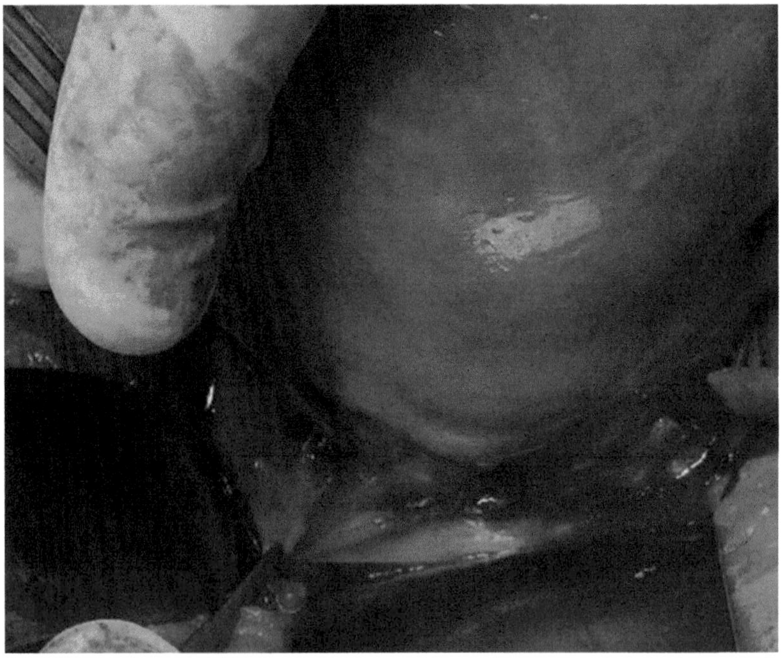

Sharp dissection has started in the midpoint (Fig. 6.1d). Bleeding has also started. Using sponge on holder to push the bladder down will lead to a lot of bleeding which can be difficult to control. In those cases where there is a history of LSCS delivery, the bladder may be densely adherent in the midline, and it might be easier to begin the dissection a bit laterally, more toward the uterines, where the uterovaginal fold may not have been opened during the LSCS.

Fig. 6.1e

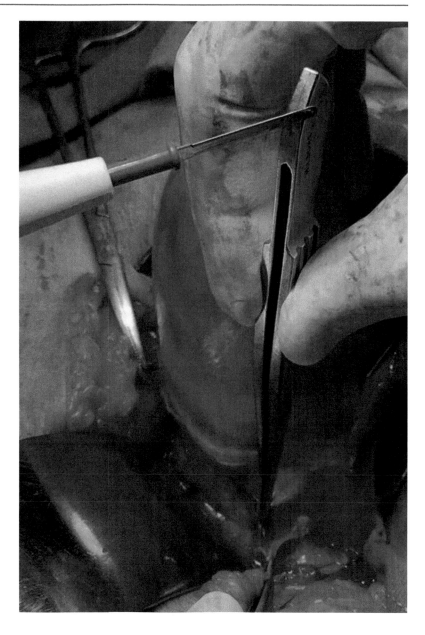

Sharp dissection is being done little by little, a small fold of tissue being held, cauterized, and then cut (Fig. 6.1e). The dissection here is being done a bit laterally, not in the midline.

In the above image, dissection is being done a bit laterally, not in the midline.

The cauterized tissue is being cut, the plane of dissection being as close to the specimen as possible (Fig. 6.1f); throughout the dissection, the assistant is holding the specimen with moderate traction in upward direction. One can appreci-

ate, the tissues are more densely adherent in the midline.

The bladder is slowly being pushed down (Fig. 6.1g). A bloodless plane has been found and the tissues- the pubocervical ligaments are being dissected.

It is now apparent that there is a long cervix (Fig. 6.1h). The bladder needs to be separated even further. The dissection is yet to begin on the other side. And it has to be done till the bladder is well below the cervix. The bladder must be pushed

Fig. 6.1f

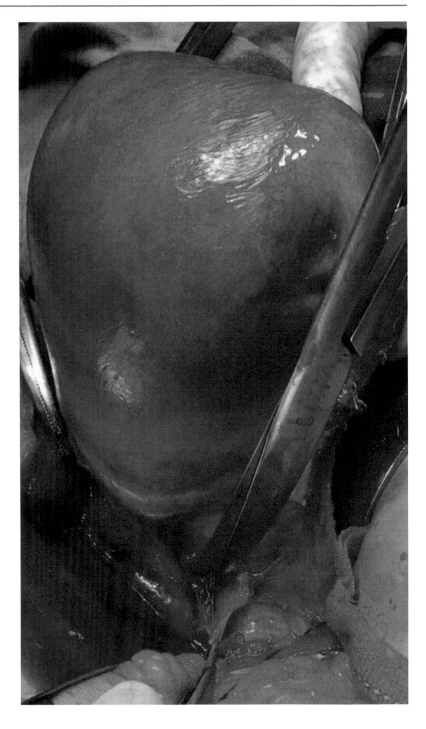

well below the cervicovaginal junction before the clamps to remove the specimen can be applied.

The dissection has begun on the opposite side (Fig. 6.1i). A small fold of tissue being held cauterized and cut as close as possible to the speci-men. A little lateral from the point of dissection is the descending cervical branch of the uterine artery. Blunt dissection when the planes are not apparent can lead to the vessels getting sheared off, leading to profuse hemorrhage.

Fig. 6.1g

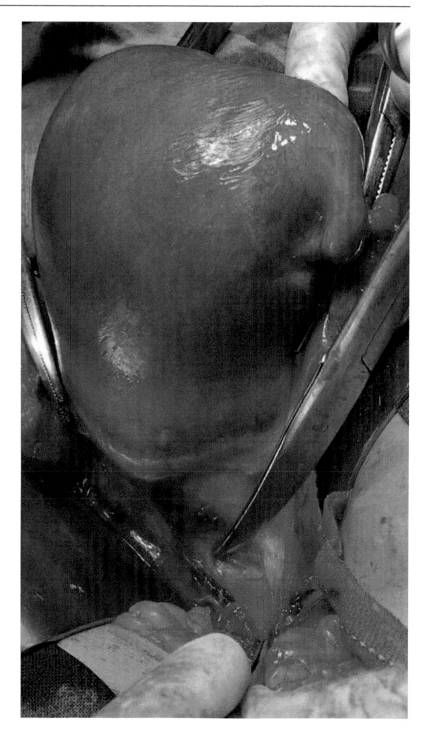

Fig. 6.1h

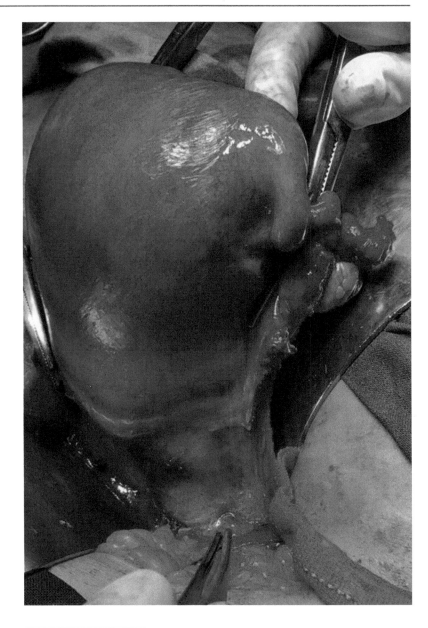

Adherent Bladder in a Case of Multiple Leiomyomas with a Large Cervical Leiomyoma (Fig. 6.2)

In Fig. 6.2, the uterovesical fold has been carefully separated and the bladder pushed down, well below the cervix.

The uterovesical fold was opened along the line of the scar of previous LSCS. The arrow is showing a faint line, the scar of previous LSCS. The space was developed by taking small chunks of tissue with a pointed forceps and cauterizing it. One must take care that cautery is applied close to the specimen, well away from bladder. Then using tissue cutting scissors, the cauterized chunk of tissue was cut. The uterovesical fold was opened in this way, till the point where the cervical vaginal junction was clearly felt. Cautery burns marks are on the specimen and not the bladder—a very important precaution. Should there be cautery burns on the bladder wall, keep the patient catheterized. Sudden appearance of blood in urine after

Fig. 6.1i

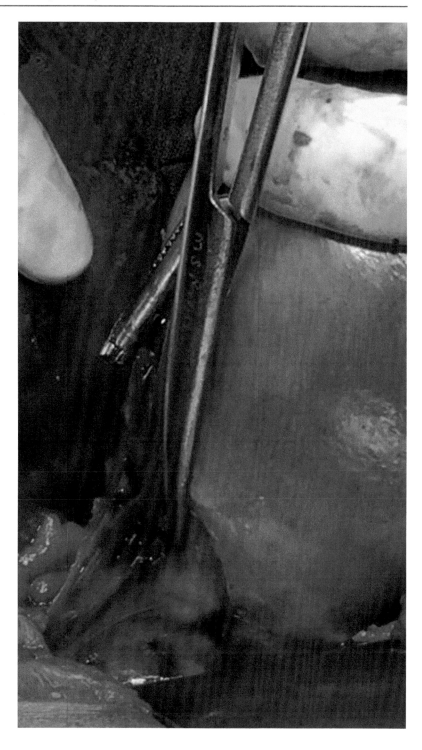

the fifth day of surgery is a sign of developing vesicovaginal fistula.

The above dissection is clean and relatively bloodless. The cervicovaginal junction was well made out in this case. But what does one do when it is not well made out?

Note: This example, that is, cervical leiomyoma, has been depicted in the next chapter in

Fig. 6.2

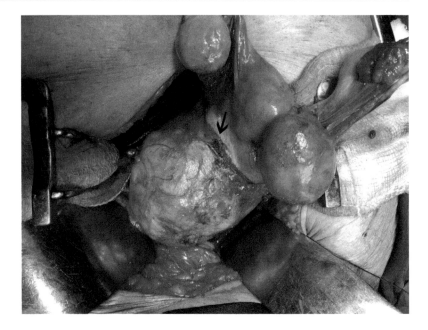

detail. Here in this chapter, this image has been shown to illustrate the neat bloodless separation of the uterovesical fold. The dissection has been done by remaining close to the specimen throughout.

How to Proceed if the Cervicovaginal Junction Cannot be Well Made Out? (Fig. 6.3a–j)

What can be done if the bladder is very densely adhered to the uterus and the cervicovaginal junction cannot be made out well? How much further down should one dissect?

One option is to ask an assistant to insert a gloved finger into the vagina from below and push the cervix up. The point where the assistant's finger is seen projecting is the cervicovaginal junction. If the bladder has been pushed well below this point, one can open the vagina and remove the specimen. Another option is to deliver the cervix posteriorly and then release the uterus out from its vaginal attachment.

Figure 6.3a shows the posterior surface of the uterus. The uterosacral ligaments are seen attached to the cervix at 5 o'clock and 7 o'clock positions as pointed out by the two arrows. Both the uterine arteries have been clamped, cut, and ligated. The

Mackenrodt's ligaments have been clamped, cut, and transfixed on both sides as shown by the stump on the left side. In many cases, the Mackenrodt's and the uterosacral ligaments cannot be taken on one single clamp because of an elongated cervix. One can clamp, cut, and transfix the uterosacrals separately. This will also help in making the uterus more mobile, since the attachment of the uterus to the sacrum has been released.

On the right lower side, one can see the ovary which is not being removed in the above case. The tip of the artery forceps is holding the stay suture taken on the round ligament (not seen in the image).

The uterosacral ligament being held with a clamp, as pointed out by the arrow (Fig. 6.3b). It is being clamped separately, not along with the Mackenrodt's ligament.

The uterosacral ligament being cut (Fig. 6.3c). One can see that only the uterosacral has been included in the clamp.

The cut uterosacral ligament being transfixed (Fig. 6.3d), this step is important for the fact that ureter can be injured during the dissection of uterosacral ligaments. The clamp has to be applied very close to the specimen. The stitch has to be taken just medial to the cut ligament.

The vagina has been opened posteriorly after the uterosacral ligaments have been clamped, cut,

Fig. 6.3a

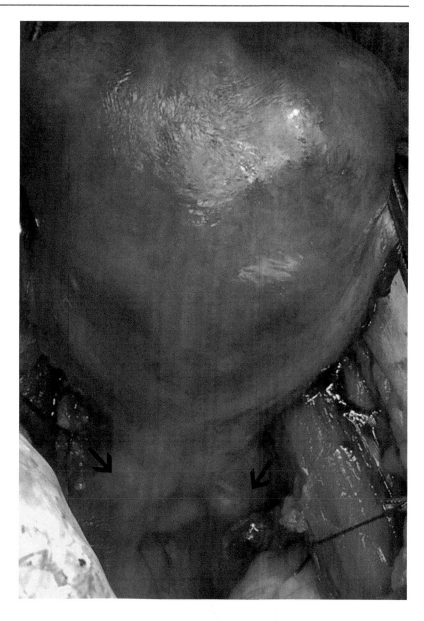

and transfixed (Fig. 6.3e). This has been done since the cervicovaginal junction was not well made out anteriorly. Injury to the bladder can be avoided by opening the vagina posteriorly. The gynecologist is excising the specimen from its vaginal attachment using cautery and has placed his finger inside the vagina as a guard. The first assistant is giving moderate upward traction to the specimen.

The specimen has been completely released from the vagina along the posterior surface (Fig. 6.3f). The cervix is being held with Allis forceps. Now the vaginal attachments have to be released anteriorly and laterally to deliver the specimen. The uterosacral stump with the stay suture can be seen in the lower end of the image, below the cervix. A closer examination of the specimen shows that the dissection has been done very close to it.

The vagina has been opened posteriorly after both the uterosacral ligaments were clamped, cut, and transfixed (Fig. 6.3g). The gynecologist's finger has been inserted into the vagina, and the specimen has been lifted using moderate traction. Cautery is being used to excise the specimen

Fig. 6.3b

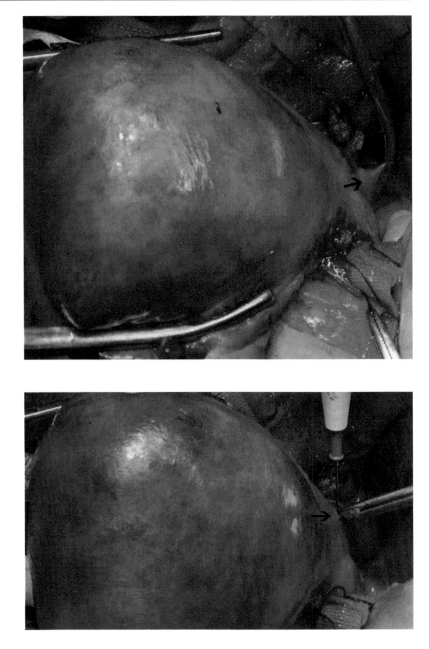

Fig. 6.3c

from the vagina with the gloved finger acting like a protective guard. Care has to be taken to be as close as possible to the cervicovaginal junction.

The specimen being removed, the posterior attachment, has been completely released; now the lateral attachment is being excised (Fig. 6.3h). The gynecologist's finger is functioning like a protective guard. The line of excision is along the cervicovagi-

nal junction. Ureters lie close to the lateral vaginal fornices, and this point is another common site where ureteric injuries occur frequently.

The specimen is being excised from the vaginal attachment anteriorly (Fig. 6.3i). The bladder is being pushed down by the Deavor's retractor. It is now apparent that the cervix is flush with vagina, thus the cervicovaginal junc-

Fig. 6.3d

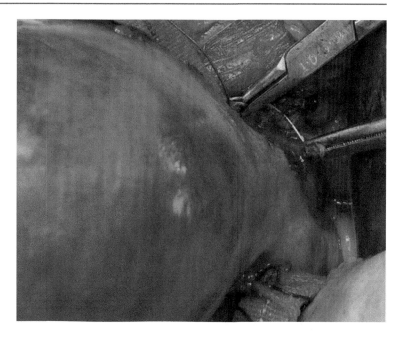

Fig. 6.3e

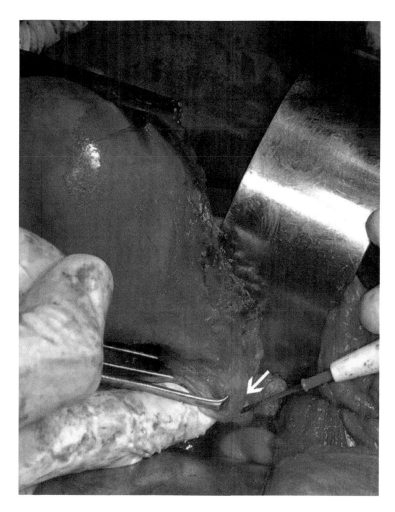

Fig. 6.3f

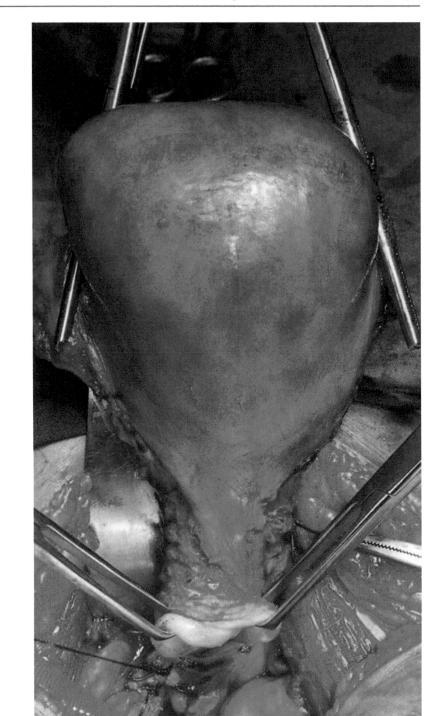

Fig. 6.3g

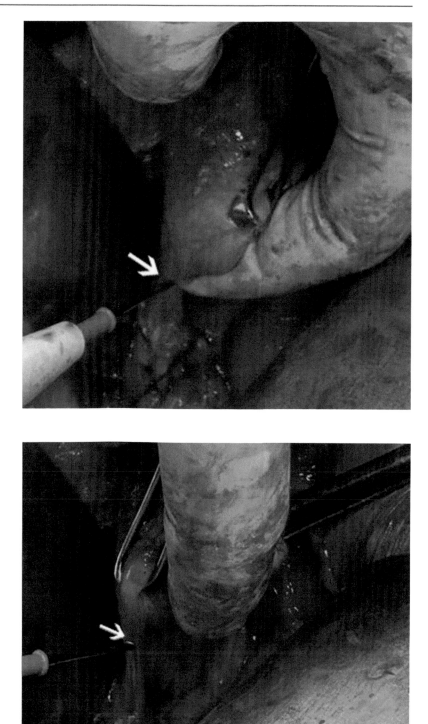

Fig. 6.3h

Fig. 6.3i

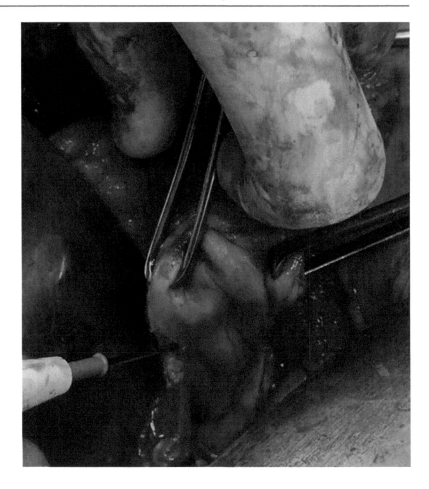

tion was not easily felt after the adherent bladder was pushed down.

The specimen has been released posteriorly and laterally on both sides, and almost along the entire length anteriorly from the vagina (Fig. 6.3j). It now needs to be released at the midpoint anteriorly. Now the specimen can be removed without any fear of injury to the bladder. While closing the vaginal vault, the vault angles can be suspended to the uterosacral pedicles to reduce the risk of vault prolapse; and small bites have to be taken along the anterior vagina making sure that the bladder tissue is not included in any of the stitches.

Fig. 6.3j

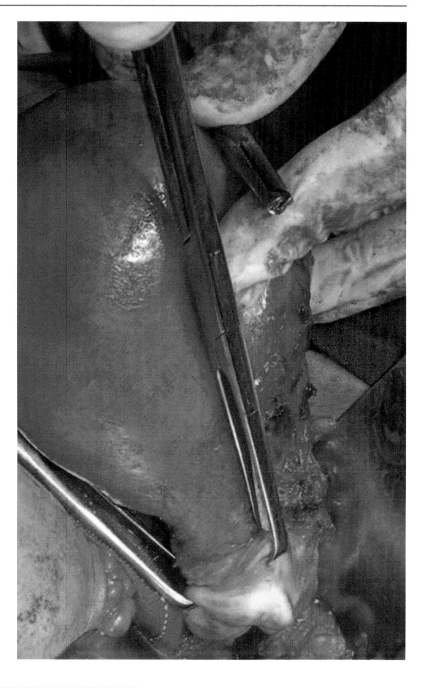

References

1. Seth S, Nagrath A. Preventing bladder injury at hysterectomy in post-cesareans. J Gynecol Womens Health. 2017;3(2):555610. https://doi.org/10.19080/JGWH.2017.03.555610.

2. Tarney CM. Bladder injury during cesarean delivery. Curr Womens Health Rev. 2013;9(2):70–6.

Endometriosis, Cervical and Broad Ligament Leiomyomas: *How to Avoid Injuries*

7

The principles of dissection are essentially same for conservative and destructive surgeries. The conservative surgery for endometriosis involves removal of the endometriotic lesions which could be densely adherent and could involve bowel, bladder, and ureter. Therefore, the same dissection techniques apply. However, myomectomy has not been considered here since it is almost always done for improving fertility or for removing symptomatic leiomyomas in younger women [1]. When hysterectomy is not desired, then there is generally no point in operating on an asymptomatic woman with leiomyoma. Asymptomatic leiomyomas should be removed when

- It is located very close to a vital organ and its further growth can make the removal more difficult and increase the risks of intraoperative injuries.
- Sudden increase in size, large size, or appearance after menopause; when exact nature of the leiomyoma/adnexal mass not certain— possibility of malignancy cannot be ruled out.
- It is causing infertility.

Multiple symptomatic leiomyomas and large leiomyomas are better treated by hysterectomy, preferably laparoscopic hysterectomy, even in young women, because if infertility is the pri-

mary complaint, then uterine artery embolization, IVF, surrogacy, etc. and not myomectomy should be considered as the first option [1]. The successful removal of leiomyomas and conception are two different issues. However, should myomectomy be done for improving fertility, the leiomyoma(s) must be removed without incising the uterine cavity or must be removed through a single incision in the uterine cavity. The risks of preterm labor, uterine rupture, placenta previa, and placenta accreta are high if the uterine cavity was opened during myomectomy [2]. Uterine artery embolization is not a good option if hysterectomy is not desired and has to be avoided at any cost, and neither is it a good option if infertility is the main complaint.

Endometriosis is a common cause of frozen pelvis [3]. Cervical and broad ligament leiomyomas are known for their proximity to the ureters, and uretric injuries are common while operating in these situations. Preoperative imaging might show hydroureters if the ureteric compression is long-standing. There could be additional challenges like densely adherent bladder due to previous LSCS, and there could also be adhesions due to previous fertility sparing/suboptimal surgery. Endometriosis can involve the rectum and may be extensive [3, 4]. If ureteric reimplantation, resection, and anastomosis of affected segment of bowel need to be done, then the surgery should be planned with a urologist and/or surgeon scrubbed in from the beginning. If infertility and not pain is the main symptom and the surgery is planned for

---

This section is written mainly considering destructive surgeries in mind, that is, hysterectomy and salpingo-oophorectomy.

© Springer Nature Singapore Pte Ltd. 2020
A. R. Podder, J. G Seshadri, *Atlas of Difficult Gynecological Surgery*,
https://doi.org/10.1007/978-981-13-8173-7_7

improving fertility, then the options of IVF and surrogacy should be discussed [1]. Surgery can guarantee permanent removal of the disease and not of fertility, since other factors like ovulation defects, tubal block, partner's fertility, etc. may also coexist.

The principles of dissection are fundamentally the same—sharp dissection.

Take a vertical incision if there has been a previous failed, suboptimal surgery. Do not directly go for a transverse incision. Use laparoscopy as a diagnostic tool to assess and then decide if the surgery can be done laparoscopically or which incision would be better for an open surgery.

Locate the ureters after dividing the round ligament. If round ligaments cannot be located due previous surgery, then hold the peritoneum on the lateral side of pelvis and open the retroperitoneal space. Locate the iliac vessels and the ureter. Take the ureter on a tape, if required. Take care not to pull the tape. At every point of dissection, check if ureter is away and is well protected. Check all the points where stitches have been taken and cautery has been applied. Are they well away from the ureter? Gently stimulate the ureter and look for peristalsis.

Separate the bowel adhesions by sharp dissection only. Make sure you do not cut the mesentery away from the bowel. Dissect along the antimesenteric side of the bowel.

At the end of the procedure, trace the small bowel from the duodenojejunal flexure to ileocaecal junction, in case of extensive endometriosis involving the bowel and if extensive dissection has been done. Check caecum, transverse colon, sigmoid, and rectum. If a bowel injury is suspected, pour copious amount of warm saline inside the peritoneal cavity and look for bubbles coming out of the submerged bowel loops. Ask an assistant to push a jet of air into the rectum and see if there are any bubbles coming out.

Now let us analyze some photographs taken during live surgery of endometriosis, cervical leiomyoma, and broad ligament leiomyoma.

Endometriosis (Fig. 7.1a–f)

The abdomen has been inadvertently opened by a transverse incision (Fig. 7.1a). The author was called after the abdomen was opened. This is a case of suspected endometriosis, and the patient had undergone one previous suboptimal surgery.

Fig. 7.1a

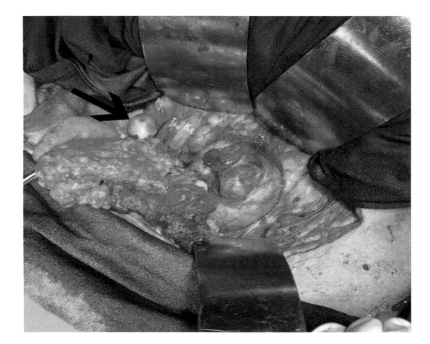

Either the abdomen should have been opened by a vertical incision, or a laparoscope should have been inserted by the open technique and the extent of disease should have been assessed. However, the surgery was accomplished without any injury to any of the vital structures.

One can see dense adhesions between the posterior uterine surface and the rectum. Also, there are dense adhesions between the omentum, pelvic organs, and the anterior abdominal wall. The omentum has been divided and the portion which is adherent to the dome of bladder is being held by an Allis forceps. The spherical structure lying between both the Deavor's retractors looks like the uterine fundus? Or is it the ovary with endometriotic cyst? Endometriosis need not present as typical chocolate cysts. It can be reddish, yellowish, or even normal pink in color [5]. However, finding chocolate cysts with the typical thick brown contents is pathognomonic of endometriosis.

Dissection has begun (Fig. 7.1b). The dense adhesions between rectum and uterus can be appreciated. The right ovary can be seen, but the left ovary is hidden and is seen partially.

The fundus is not visible, probably removed during previous surgery (Fig. 7.1b). There were no records as to what was removed during previous surgery.

The first step in such situations is to locate the ureter lest it gets damaged (Fig. 7.1c). The arrow is pointing to the point in the lateral wall of the pelvis, where one can find some space to lift a fold of peritoneum. This will be opened to gain access to the retroperitoneal space to locate the left ureter. As one can see, there is no identifiable round ligament. The round ligament is the most consistent landmark in a female pelvis, and a stay suture can be taken on it. It can be divided and the retroperitoneal space opened. The ureter can be found along the medial fold of the broad ligament. But when there is no recognizable round ligament, one can hold a fold of peritoneum laterally and open it to gain access to the retroperitoneum as is being done above.

The same step being done on the right side, lifting a fold of peritoneum in the right lateral pelvic wall to open the retroperitoneal space on the right side in order to locate the right ureter (Fig. 7.1d).

Something ruptured! Fortunately it is not fecal matter, it is "chocolate," an endometrioma, which has ruptured (Fig. 7.1e). This can seed in the pouch of Douglas and can cause persistent symptoms later. A thorough irrigation of the entire peritoneal cavity is a must at the end of the surgery to flush out all the remnant endometriotic tissue [6].

Fig. 7.1b

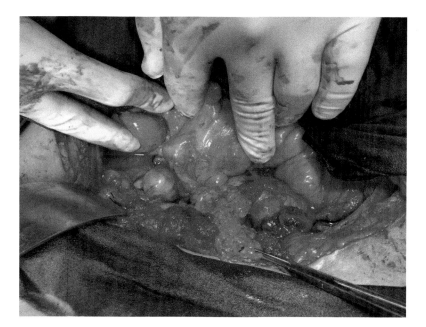

Fig. 7.1c

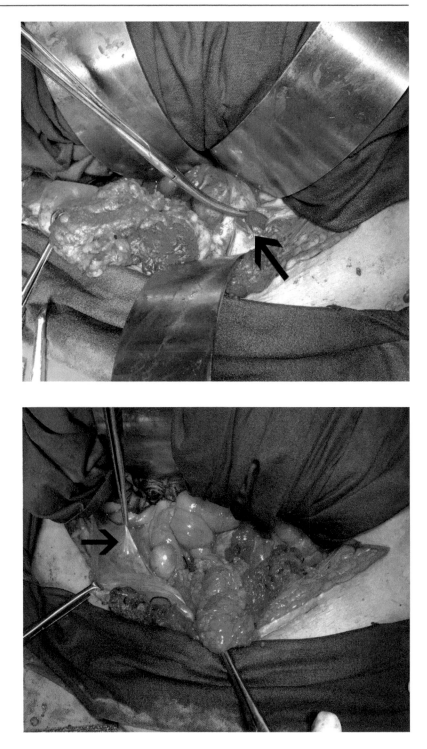

Fig. 7.1d

The ureter has been finally located (Fig. 7.1f). One can take it on a tape, and this will help lateralizing it. Once the ureters are safely out of the way, hysterectomy can be performed safely. In Fig. 7.1f, it is now obvious that there is a uterus in situ. Probably during the previous surgery, only some chocolate cysts were removed, and the uterus was left in situ. The Babcock forceps is holding the right cornu of the uterus. Also, one can see

Fig. 7.1e

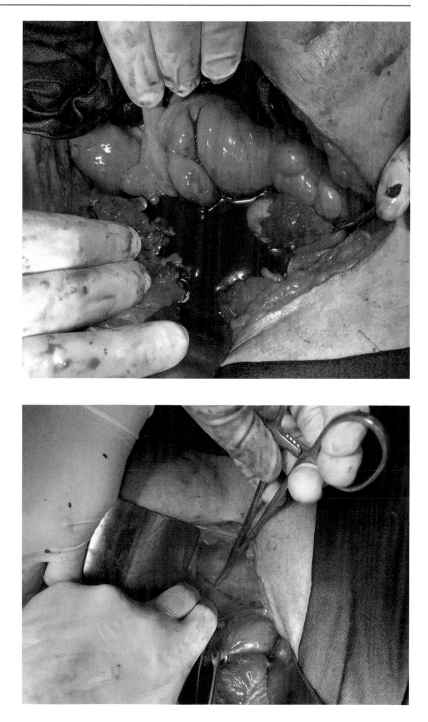

Fig. 7.1f

that the rectum (as can be appreciated from the Fig. 7.1a, b, the rectum was densely adherent to the posterior surface of the uterus) has been separated from the posterior uterine surface by sharp dissection.

Cervical Leiomyoma (Fig. 7.2a–e)

A case of multiple leiomyomas (Fig. 7.2a), the photo has been captured from above. The umbilicus is seen down and the symphysis pubis is

Fig. 7.2a

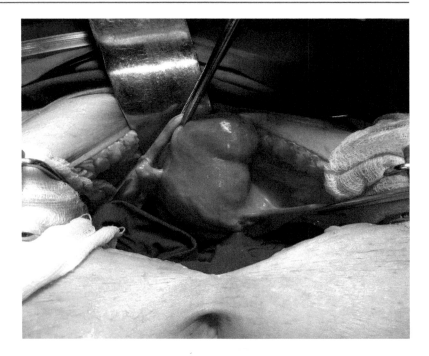

Fig. 7.2b

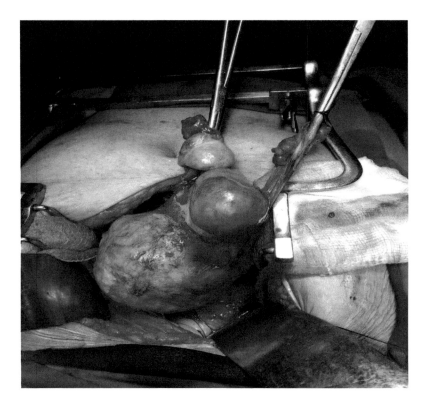

Fig. 7.2c

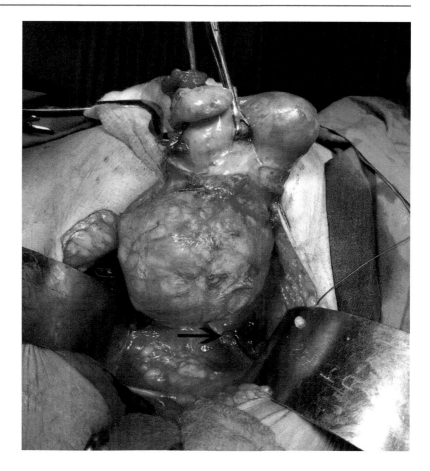

above the incision. The round ligaments will now be divided to locate the ureter. There is a large cervical leiomyoma in addition to a fundal leiomyoma.

Broad ligament and cervical leiomyomas are known for their proximity to the ureter, and this fact has to be kept in mind while doing myomectomy and hysterectomy.

Uterovesical fold has been well separated and the bladder pushed well below the cervix (Fig. 7.2b). Cautery burn marks sustained during the separation of bladder are seen on the cervix. Let the specimen sustain injuries and burns but not bladder, ureter, or the bowel!

In Fig. 7.2c, the arrow is pointing toward the descending branch of uterine artery which has been ligated using black silk. One can imagine the bleeding that would have occurred if the bladder had been pushed down with a "peanut" or "sponge on holder." It would have been profuse and would have also obscured the operating field. "Attempts to secure hemostasis" is the step during which most of the ureteric injuries are known to occur. The other steps being the clamping of infundibulopelvic ligament, uterine artery, uterosacral ligament, and the vaginal vault angles; the ureters lie close to these structures and can get injured if clamps are not placed close to the specimen, or if there is a large adnexal mass, cervical/broad ligament leiomyoma wherein the ureter is situated very close to the specimen and is more vulnerable to injury than usual [7, 8].

Fig. 7.2d

Fig. 7.2e

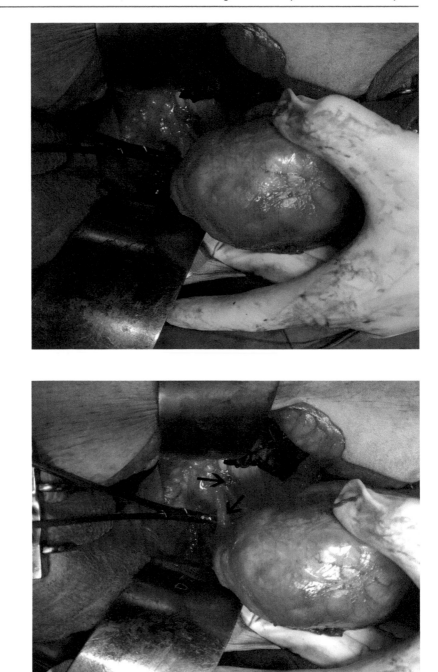

The ureter has been located (Fig. 7.2d). This view is from the top. The right-angled forceps has been passed under the ureter. One can appreciate how close it is to the specimen. A cursory glance may result in a ureteric injury, especially while clamping the uterine arteries and uterosacral ligaments or while suturing the vaginal vault angles.

The arrow pointing down shows the ureter with a right-angled forceps under it (Fig. 7.2e). The upper arrow is pointing to uterine artery which has been cut and cauterized making sure that the ureter is away and will not get damaged by cautery. Now, one can apply the uterosacral clamps being sure that the ureter will not get included in it.

Broad Ligament Leiomyoma
(Fig. 7.3a–d)

A broad ligament leiomyoma (Fig. 7.3a), this was an unexpected finding on the operating table, not suggested on clinical examination or pre-operative imaging. The space is not sufficient; an additional assistant has been called to scrub in just to hold the retractors. Rectus abdominis muscle has been cut transversely on both sides to facilitate better exposure. Fortunately, there are no adhesions. A stay suture had been taken on the round ligament on one side, and the fold of broad ligament will be opened to locate the ureter and make sure it is away from the operating field.

The folds of the broad ligament have been opened (Fig. 7.3b). The broad ligament leiomyoma is seen as a separate mass from the uterine fundus. It can be removed as a separate entity. This will free up some space and make rest of the surgery easier. But a word of caution: what if the leiomyoma is malignant—a sarcoma? Removing piecemeal or using a myoma screw during laparoscopy can lead to peritoneal seeding. Sarcomas are known for their very high rate of recurrence [9, 10]. Avoid splitting or morcellating the uterus, if the previous imaging reports show that the leiomyoma has suddenly increased in size or if the patient is postmenopausal, or if it appears unusually fleshy and vascular.

Similarly, while doing a hysterectomy (which could be abdominal, vaginal, or laparoscopic) for a case of complex atypical hyperplasia of the endometrium, one must keep in mind that there could be a coexisting foci of carcinoma endometrium which might have been missed in endometrial sampling or D&C. There could be adenocarcinoma of the endometrium in upto 40% of the hysterectomies performed for complex atypical hyperplasia. Thus the gynecologist must cut open the specimen after removing it intact, to look for any growth in the endometrium and gross signs of myometrial invasion. The patient and her relatives should be informed that a staging and completion of surgery would be necessary if the histopathology report turns out to be positive for carcinoma endometrium [11].

As mentioned before, one must either open through a vertical incision or preferably insert a laparoscope and then decide—laparoscopy or laparotomy. This was another case where the author was called after the abdomen was opened. Fortunately it was possible to accomplish the hysterectomy without problems.

The broad ligament leiomyoma has been completely separated/shelled out from the broad ligament (Fig. 7.3c). It has not been morcellated

Fig. 7.3a

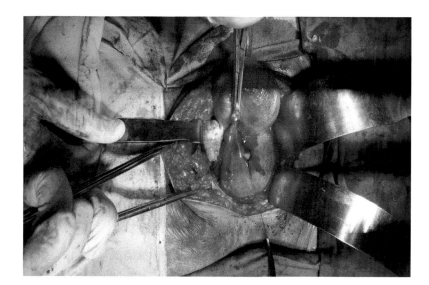

Fig. 7.3b

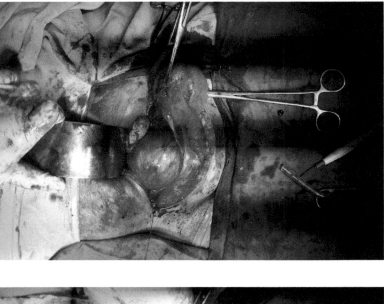

Fig. 7.3c

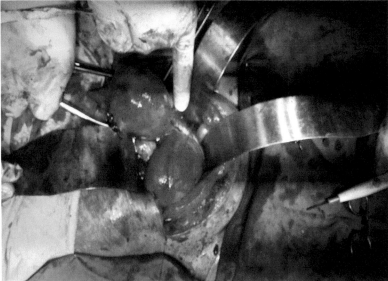

in situ. The intention is to remove the specimen as one mass.

The ureter and the uterine artery must be below the leiomyoma, could well be just below it. It is important to locate the ureter before applying clamps on the side of the broad ligament leiomyoma.

The ureter has finally been located (Fig. 7.3d). This image shows the assistant holding the specimen with both hands; it is hidden inside his palms. One hand of the operating gynecologist is retracting the bowels and preventing them from falling into the operating field. The patient has been given a head low position. Sometimes,

patients start pushing toward the end of surgery when the effect of spinal anesthesia is beginning to wear off. There is a stay suture on the round ligament, held by an artery forceps. The ureter is fortunately far down below. It must be somewhere near the arrow pointing downwards. The arrow pointing up is pointing at the stitch that has been taken on the specimen, to ligate the descending branch of uterine artery. From the above image, one can appreciate that the cervix is elongated and thin like a stalk, whereas the fundus along with the broad ligament leiomyoma are quite big in size.

Fig. 7.3d

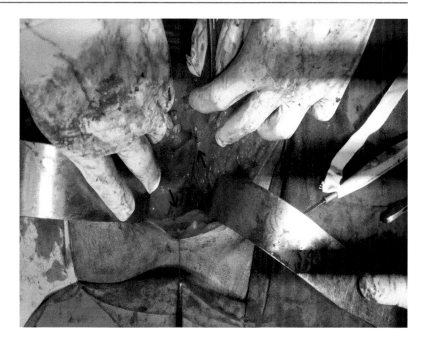

References

1. Rakotomahenina H, Rajaonarison J, Wong L, Brun JL. Myomectomy: technique and current indications. Minerva Ginecol. 2017;69(4):357–69.
2. Kim HS, et al. Uterine rupture in pregnancies following myomectomy: a multicenter case series. Obstet Gynecol Sci. 2016;59(6):454–62.
3. Mohling SI, Elkattah R, Furr RS. Endometriosis: tools for the frozen pelvis. J Minim Invasive Gynecol. 2015;22(6):S139.
4. De La Hera-Lazara, et al. Radical surgery for endometriosis: analysis of quality of life and surgical procedure. Clin Med Insights Women's Health. 2016;9:7–11.
5. Stegmann BJ, et al. Using location, color, size, and depth to characterize and identify endometriosis lesions in a cohort of 133 women. Fertil Steril. 2008;89(6):1632–6.
6. Llewellyn-Bennett, et al. Iatrogenic endometriosis of the vaginal vault following a total laparoscopic hysterectomy. West Lond Med J. 2010;2(4):1–4.
7. Engelsgjerd JS, LaGrange CA. Ureteral injury. Treasure Island, FL: StatPearls Publishing; 2018. Last Update: October 27.
8. Burks FN, Santucci RA. Management of iatrogenic ureteral injury. Ther Adv Urol. 2014;6(3):115–24.
9. El-Khalfaoui K, Bois A, Heitz, Kurzeder C, Sehouli J, Harter P. Current and future options in the management and treatment of uterine sarcoma. Ther Adv Med Oncol. 2014;6(1):21–8.
10. Liu H, Zhu Y, Zhang G, Wang C, Li C, Shi Y. Laparoscopic surgery on broken points for uterine sarcoma in the early stage decrease prognosis. Sci Rep. 2016;6:31229.
11. Trimble CL, et al. Concurrent endometrial carcinoma in women with a biopsy diagnosis of atypical endometrial hyperplasia: a gynecologic oncology group study. Cancer. 2006;106:812–9.

Pelvic Abscess: *Surgical Drainage and Inevitable Problems*

8

Finding pus in the abdomen and pelvis can be a surprise finding on table. Adnexal mass, torsion of a subserosal fibroid or ovarian tumor, appendicitis, etc. are conditions which can present in a similar manner and can lead to delay in the diagnosis of pelvic abscess [1, 2].

Sometimes pelvic abscess can be a confident preoperative diagnosis. Diabetics with history of poor glycemic control, history of PID, lack of asepsis during uterine evacuation or during delivery, are known causes of pelvis abscess [1, 2]. There could be fever, abdominal pain, and tenderness. Leukocytosis will always be present, unless inappropriate antibiotic treatment has been given.

So, whenever the diagnosis is uncertain, one must either take a vertical incision or must put a laparoscope and see. Colpotomy or image-guided aspiration is confirmatory; finding pus on aspiration is diagnostic of an abscess inside the peritoneal cavity, but should colpotomy be used to treat pelvic abscess? Colpotomy can only drain pus collected in the pouch of Douglas and not of the loculated pus elsewhere in the peritoneal cavity. Also, the rectum may be adherent to the posterior uterine surface, and colpotomy in such a situation may result in rectal injury [3]. Thus it is better to open and see and drain everything out.

There could be locules of pus even under the diaphragm and sub-hepatic space. The bowel loops will be agglutinated to each other if the pus has spread beyond the pelvis, and the omentum ("Policeman of the Abdomen") would have contained the pus. So one can expect the bowel walls to be inflamed and every effort has to be made to avoid injury. The results of repair on an inflamed bowel will obviously be very poor.

When pus is seen pouring out, take samples for culture, and then irrigate the abdominopelvic cavity with copious amounts of saline. Suction the collected fluid, taking care not to traumatize any organ with the suction cannula. Even gentle rubbing movements on the bowel can lead to a bowel rent. Use sharp dissection to separate the flimsy bowel adhesions. Divide the omentum which would have localized the pus, release all the locules of pus and inflammatory fluid. Examine the paracolic gutters, sub-diaphragmatic spaces, and the under surface of the liver. Gently break all the locules of pus, and release the collected fluid. Never forget to gently probe the pouch of Douglas. The pouch of Douglas being the most dependent part of the peritoneal cavity will have collected pus, which could be in encysted locules. Do not use force, lest the rectum gets damaged, and colostomy becomes necessary. If the diagnosis has been delayed for any reason, the flimsy adhesion will start getting organized making their release even more difficult and bowels are then more prone to injury.

Never perform a hysterectomy or any destructive procedure in the presence of pus. There will be lot of edema, induration, and planes will not be well delineated. The chances of ureteric and other vital organ injuries are high. Just drain the pus and remove all the necrotic material, thoroughly irrigate the entire peritoneal cavity with copious amount of saline and close. Before closing, trace

© Springer Nature Singapore Pte Ltd. 2020
A. R. Podder, J. G Seshadri, *Atlas of Difficult Gynecological Surgery*,
https://doi.org/10.1007/978-981-13-8173-7_8

the entire small intestine from duodenojejunal flexure to the ileocecal junction. Check the caecum, transverse, sigmoid, and rectum for any injuries. If there are any bands which are still intact, gently break them; use sharp dissection if the bands are getting organized and do not separate easily. If the bands and purulent flakes get organized, it can lead to intestinal obstruction [4]. Do not leave agglutinated loops of bowel unattended on grounds that the loops appear intact; patient may have vomiting and subacute bowel obstruction in the immediate postoperative period itself. The author has an experience of a case where the patient had to be taken for reexploration because pus reappeared in the drain on the third postoperative day. On table, one large locule of pus was still found intact. In a hurry to finish the case, one locule was overlooked and had not been drained.

As a rule of thumb, the author prefers closing cases of pelvic abscess (probably the only condition in gynecology where there is a dirty/contaminated wound) by delayed primary closure [5, 6].

In this method, the peritoneum is closed, followed by rectus sheath. The author does not prefer mass closure for vertical incisions because should the suture give way at any point, it will result in burst abdomen [7]. But if the peritoneum and the rectus sheath are closed separately, even if the rectus sheath suture gives way (let us say due to tissue necrosis and infection), there will be an intact peritoneum that will prevent burst abdomen. However, if factors which raise the intra-abdominal pressure like coughing, vomiting, straining, etc. are not controlled in the postoperative period, then the risk of burst abdomen is very high irrespective of the type of closure.

The skin is not closed. The wound is packed with gauze soaked in povidone iodine and changed daily. The skin is closed after anemia, dyselectrolytemia, and hypoproteinemia have been corrected by blood and albumin transfusions, and diabetes if present is also brought under control [8]. This is usually after a week. The patient would have passed stools and would have tolerated soft diet by then.

Delayed primary closure was widely used during the pre-antibiotic era, but now with growing antibiotic resistance, it is time this approach is adopted more often in situations when the possibility of wound gape is high or almost certain. This method does not reduce the incidence of incisional hernia and late intestinal obstruction due to adhesions, but certainly reduces hospital stay, treatment costs, and the use of antibiotics. The question of wound gape does not arise since the closure is done only after control and correction of associated risk factors (like anemia, hypoproteinemia, and diabetes mellitus), and after healthy granulation tissue has formed all along the wound. Delayed primary closure should not be confused with open abdomen. Open abdomen is a defect created intentionally by not closing the incision after completion of surgery; or the abdomen is opened or reopened out of concern that the patient is developing abdominal compartment syndrome.

In delayed primary closure, the rectus sheath is closed; it is the skin closure which is deferred by a few days. The wound is dressed daily with gauze soaked in povidone iodine. This improves blood supply by hygroscopic action. Also, the act of draining pus by releasing all adhesions and braking of locules will lead to bacteremia in the immediate postoperative period. The chances of wound dehiscence will be high.

By deferring the closure of skin by a week, the chances of wound healing would have greatly improved on account of better blood supply to the wound margins and control of risk factors.

Now let us study some photographs taken during live surgery of cases of pelvic abscess. The photographs are grouped in the following sequence—precautions while opening the peritoneum, separating the loops of bowel and releasing the bands, entering the pelvis and draining locules of pus, looking for hidden pockets and locules, examining and checking for injuries before closure, and finally delayed primary closure of the abdomen.

Opening the Abdomen in a Case of Pelvic Abscess (Figs. 8.1, 8.2, 8.3, 8.4, 8.5, 8.6, and 8.7a, b)

In situations where pelvic abscess is suspected or is certain preoperatively, look at the peritoneum before opening it (Fig. 8.1). It is edematous and bulging. One can be sure that there will be significant collection in the peritoneal cavity. One

Fig. 8.1

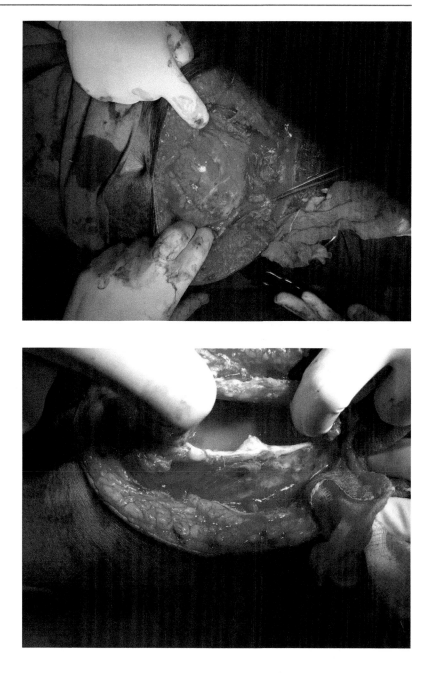

Fig. 8.2

can expect bowels to be floating in the collected fluid and may even be adhered to the parietal peritoneum underneath. Open with great care lest the bowel gets torn.

Pus immediately below the peritoneum (Fig. 8.2), collect a sample for culture and sensitivity.

Figure 8.3 is an image from another case. The peritoneum has been opened. Purulent flakes can be

seen and appreciated. The inflammatory fluid is seen pouring out. Avoid sticking the suction cannula deep inside. Bowel walls could be very friable and can get torn even by a slight jerk. Dip the suction cannula into the pool of fluid, so that the tip is visible. Take care to ensure that the omentum or the bowel wall do not get sucked into the cannula and get injured.

Figure 8.4 is another example of a pelvic abscess. Peritoneum has been opened taking care

Fig. 8.3

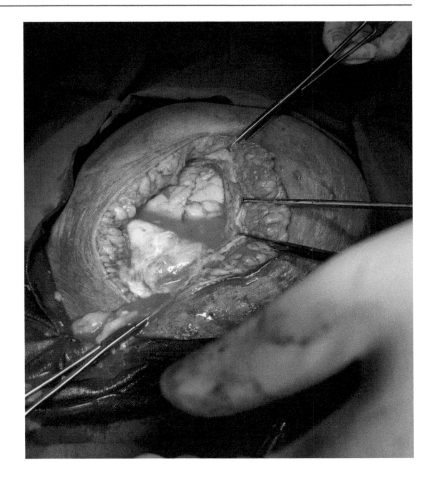

not to injure any structure. The incision length may not be enough. Extend the incision, and drain the collected fluid with the help of a suction cannula. Avoid inserting the tip of the suction cannula deep into the collection. The tip of the cannula must be visible while suctioning. There could be an inflamed friable organ deep inside the collected fluid that can get damaged by rough movements of the cannula .

The edematous loops of intestine are seen directly under the peritoneum (Fig. 8.5). The peritoneum has been opened with care. The bowel loops are agglutinated to one another and the abdominal wall. One has to gently release them lest the bands get organized and cause intestinal obstruction later.

In Fig. 8.6, the peritoneum is being opened with great care; pus is seen inside, and one must

expect inflamed bowels and pelvic organs and must proceed with caution.

Pus is getting organized and the bowels have become adherent to the overlying parietal peritoneum (Fig. 8.7a).

In Figs. 8.2, 8.3, and 8.4 one can see there is a lot of fluid in the abdominal cavity. This in a way protects the bowel from getting injured during opening of the peritoneum. The bowels by virtue of floating in the collected fluid will get pushed away if subjected to some force during opening of the peritoneum. Figure 8.7a is from a patient who was obese and diabetic, and the patient had presented late. One can see that the peritoneum has not been fully opened yet, but it is obvious that there is a lot of pus inside. The omentum can be seen forming a cake. The small intestine loop with purulent flakes can be seen below, and it is stuck

Fig. 8.4

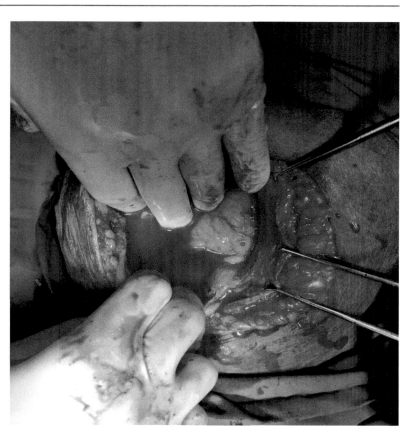

Fig. 8.5

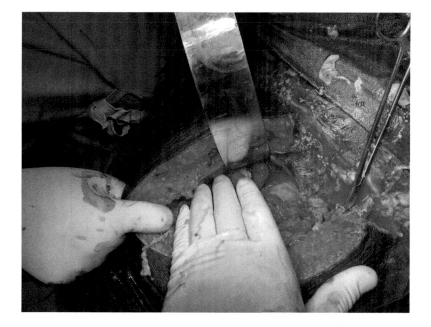

Fig. 8.6

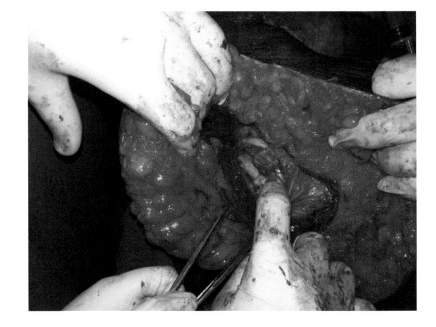

to the overlying peritoneum. Operating on a case of pelvic abscess means pausing at every step to carefully check what is there, and then proceeding again with caution. Injuries are almost always due to lack of caution, unlike let us say endometriosis where let us say resection anastomosis of affected bowel segment is intentionally performed to remove every visible trace of the disease.

Look carefully, the arrow is pointing toward the loops of small intestine which are right below the peritoneum (Fig. 8.7b). It is evident that the bowel loops are stuck to the overlying peritoneum and to each other because of flimsy adhesions and purulent flakes. Gently release the bands with tissue-cutting scissors and avoid forcefully separating the adherent structures. Obesity and the problems one can expect with regard to wound healing can also be appreciated.

Thick Reddish Brown Pus! (Fig. 8.8)

Thick reddish brownish pus pouring out after the locule has been broken (Fig. 8.8). The omentum which helps containing the pus can be seen below the gynecologist's hand.

Inflamed Bowels (Fig. 8.9)

The loops of intestine are seen agglutinated to each other and to the pelvic side walls by purulent flakes (Fig. 8.9). They will need to be broken down gently.

Pelvic Abscess can Present as Subacute Intestinal Obstruction (Fig. 8.10)

Inflammatory fluid pouring out with purulent flakes; edematous loops of small intestine are edematous and distended with gas (Fig. 8.10); there must be a band which is compressing the intestine. Hence, the part of the intestine above the obstructing band is distended, and the segment distal to the obstructing band is collapsed.

Loops of Intestine Covered with Purulent Flakes (Fig. 8.11)

Gentle separation of the loops and mesenteric folds is required (Fig. 8.11). Remember the intestines are edematous and prone for injury. If a

Fig. 8.7a

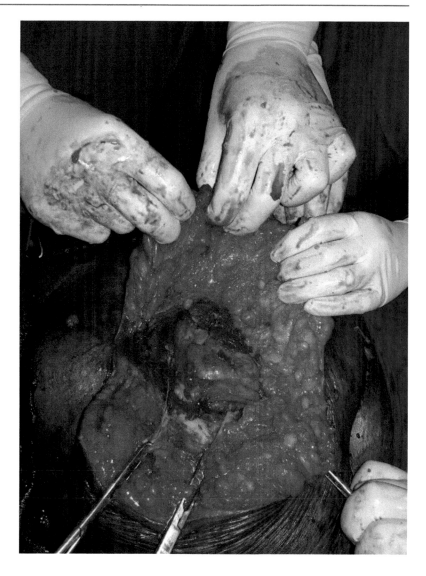

horizontal mesenteric tear occurs, it might lead to blood supply of the involved segment to get cut off. The importance of thorough irrigation of the entire peritoneal cavity before closure with drains can be appreciated from the above image.

Gently Separating the Agglutinated Loops of Intestine (Fig. 8.12)

Purulent flakes are covering the bowel loops, and the fact that bowel loops are stuck to one another can be appreciated (Fig. 8.12). The bands are getting organized. Use sharp dissection if necessary.

Even a small jerk with the little finger can rip two adherent loops, causing a rent or can tear the mesentery.

Adhesions Getting Organized
(Fig. 8.13a, b)

The adhesions over the loops of intestine are getting organized (Fig. 8.13a). The patient was referred very late; she had a history of fever with chills for more than a week and had clinical symptoms suggestive of intestinal obstruction. She was admitted under the Department of

Fig. 8.7b

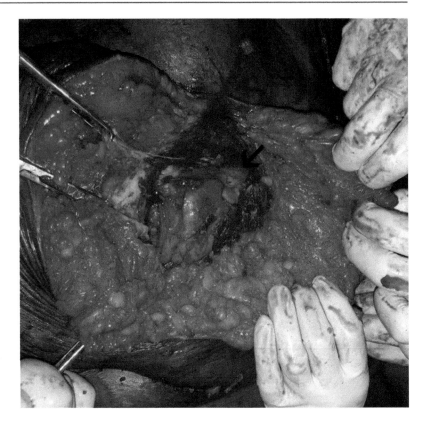

Obstetrics and Gynecology because she was a puerpera. If one observes a bit closely, the inverted T incision can be appreciated. The patient underwent an LSCS through a Pfannenstiel incision, and now a vertical incision has been taken for the drainage of pus.

The patient had received prolonged antibiotic treatment for fever. The decision to do an emergency exploratory laparotomy was taken when the imaging report showed significant collection in the peritoneal cavity. Image-guided aspiration showed straw-colored fluid with high WBC counts.

The loops of small intestine have been separated (Fig. 8.13b). The uterine fundus is now exposed, and subinvolution is evident. The pouch of Douglas needs to be explored for hidden pockets of pus. The inflamed intestines plastered with thick purulent flakes can be appreciated, but fortunately they are not damaged. They are pink and have no bluish purplish patches which are suggestive of bowel ischemia.

Entering the Pelvis (Figs. 8.14, 8.15, and 8.16)

The pelvis has finally been approached after separating the small intestines (Fig. 8.14). The purulent flakes can be seen. Now the paracolic gutters and the pouch of Douglas will have to be explored and cleared of any collected pus.

The ovary is seen intact, but loops of intestine need to be separated to gain access to pouch of Douglas (Fig. 8.15). There could be more hidden pockets of pus in the paracolic gutters and in pouch of Douglas.

The incision taken in this patient is a transverse incision. This patient is puerpera who underwent an LSCS a few days before. So it makes sense to first open the abdomen through the LSCS incision which anyway is showing sign of dehiscence. Should there be a need to explore the entire peritoneal cavity, then a vertical inci-

Fig. 8.8

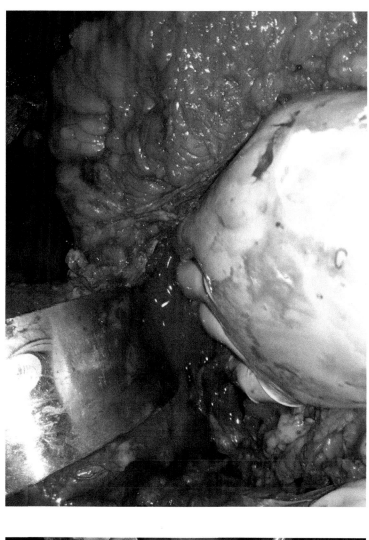

Fig. 8.9

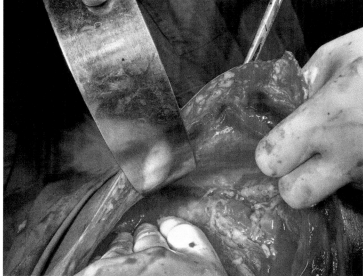

Fig. 8.10

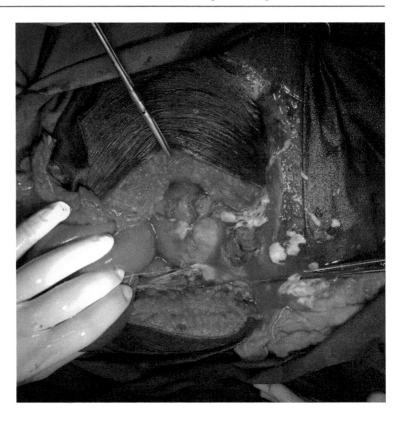

Fig. 8.11

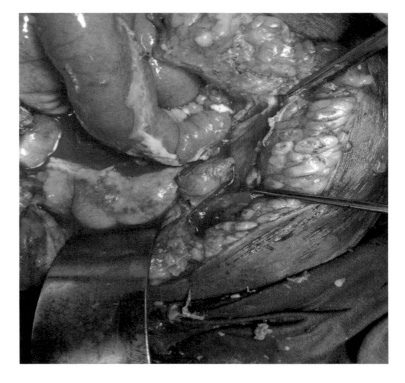

Fig. 8.12

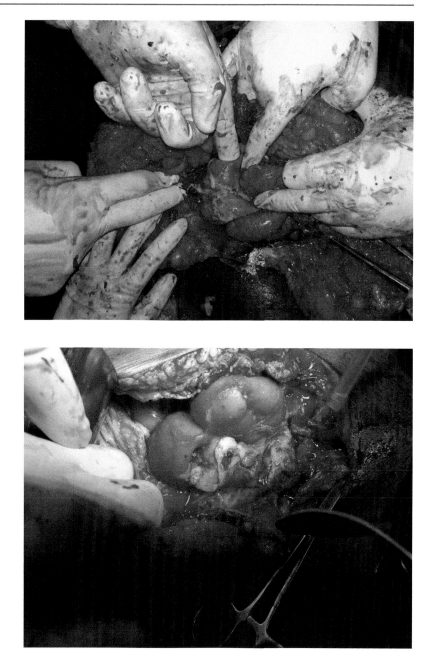

Fig. 8.13a

sion must be taken which will result in the patient having an inverted T scar.

Thick purulent flakes have plastered the pelvic viscera; sharp dissection is the rule (Fig. 8.16). There could be a lot of pus hidden in the pouch of Douglas, so one has to separate the bands gently in order to drain all the collected pus and fluid.

Pus in the Pelvis (Figs. 8.17, 8.18, 8.19, and 8.20)

Pelvic abscess in a patient who underwent an LSCS some days back (Fig. 8.17), purulent flakes on the uterine sutures can be seen. Uterine subinvolution is also apparent.

Fig. 8.13b

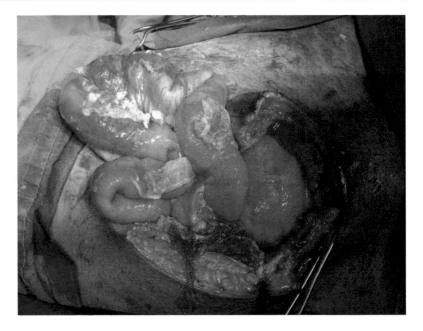

Fig. 8.14

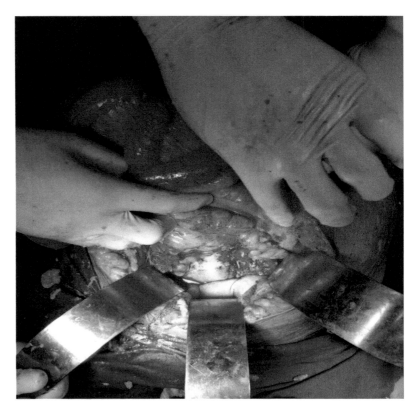

Fig. 8.15

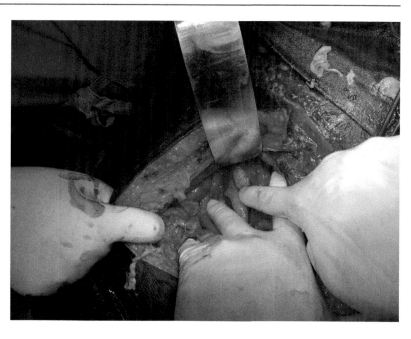

Fig. 8.16

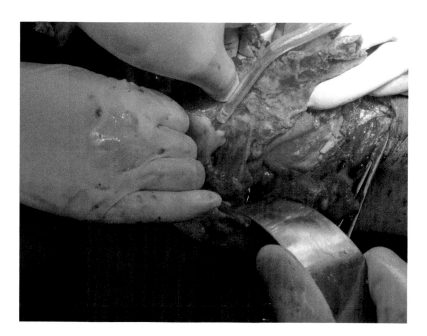

Thick Yellow Green Pus

Thick yellow green pus is pouring out of the uterus (Fig. 8.18)—a sample being collected for culture and sensitivity. The operating gynecologist has held the fundus of the uterus with his right hand between his thumb and fingers and is holding the syringe with his left hand. One may not be able to appreciate that the structure being held is actually the uterus. A small nick has been made on the anterior surface of the uterus which was soft and bulging to release the pus.

The uterus has not become a pelvic organ yet, and there is subinvolution of the uterus due to

Fig. 8.17

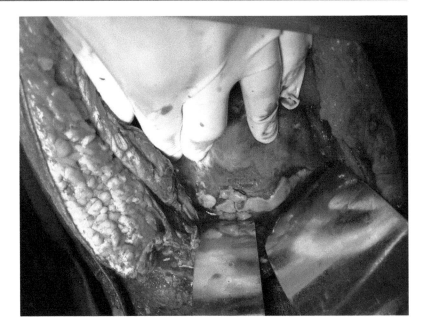

Fig. 8.18

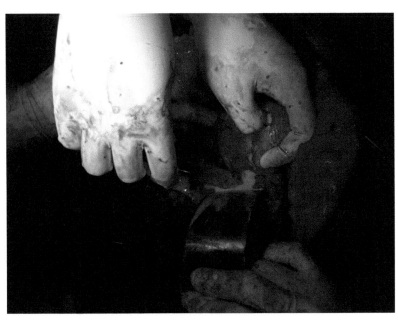

infection (Fig. 8.19). Thick yellow pus is seen pouring out of the uterine fundus.

Pus and Flakes in the Adnexa

When there are flakes over the uterus and adnexa, no attempt should be made to excise it (Fig. 8.20). Gently remove what comes off easily. Thorough lavage should be given to remove all the necrotic materials and debris. The risk of future intestinal

obstruction and chronic pelvic pain due to post-operative adhesions can occur in future.

The Under Surface of Liver
(Figs. 8.21, 8.22, 8.23, and 8.24)

The under surface of liver is now being examined (Fig. 8.21). The main part of the procedure—draining the pus in the pelvis—has been accomplished and a thorough lavage has been given.

Fig. 8.19

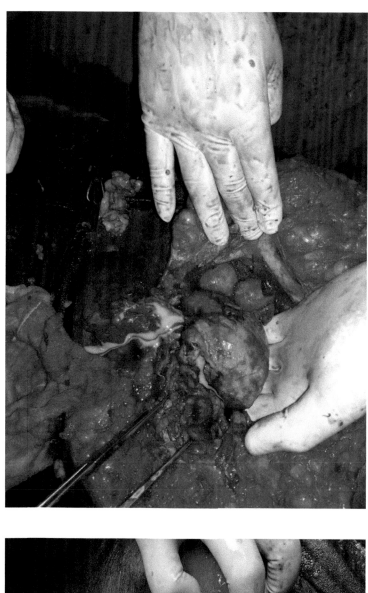

Fig. 8.20

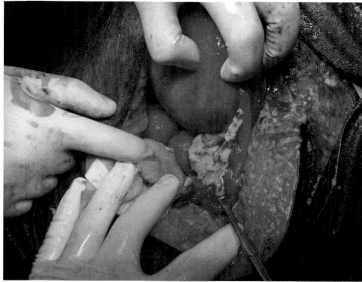

Fig. 8.21

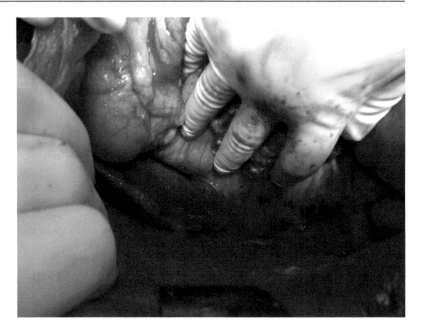

Fig. 8.22

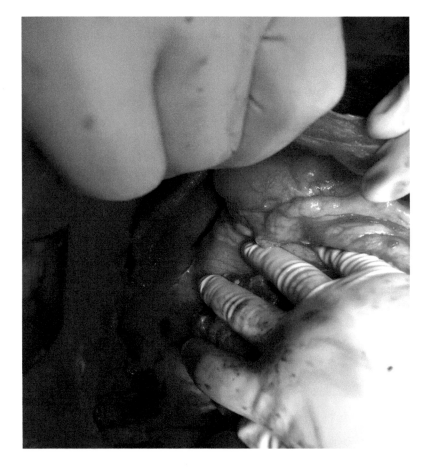

Fig. 8.23

Fig. 8.24

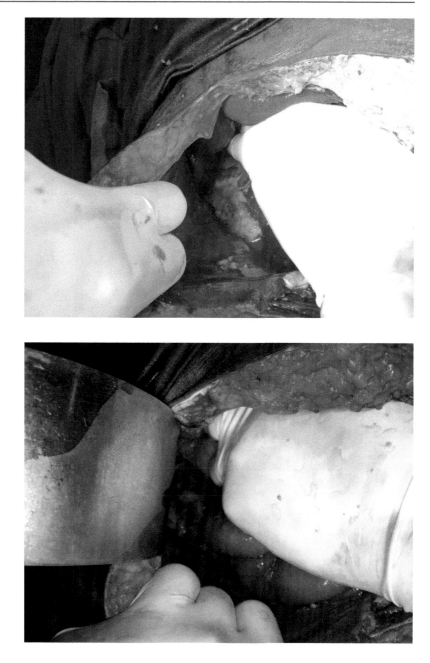

But before closing the abdomen, just look for any hidden collections and locules elsewhere in the peritoneal cavity. If present, they should be gently broken and the collection should be drained.

Collection and purulent flakes in the undersurface of liver can be appreciated (Fig. 8.22). Avoid traumatizing the liver surface with the suction cannula. Bleeding if it occurs will be torrential and very difficult to control given the inflammation present. Liver even in normal situations is a soft organ that can get easily traumatized by a forceful jerk.

There are a lot of purulent flakes in the undersurface of liver in this case (Fig. 8.23). The area should be flushed with a generous amount of saline and irrigation suction should be done till most of the necrotic materials get washed off. Remember not to forcefully peel out what is stuck. Never scrape the surface of liver with the suction cannula with the intention of peeling the purulent flakes. Should bleeding start in this region, it will be very profuse and very difficult to control.

A locule in the undersurface of liver; it needs to be gently broken down/punctured to release the pocket of pus (Fig. 8.24). One must do it very carefully without injuring the liver surface or parenchyma.

Examine the Entire Bowel Before Closing the Abdomen with Drain in Situ (Fig. 8.25)

After draining all the pus, the entire small intestine has been traced from duodenojejunal flexure, and it is intact (Fig. 8.25). A few purulent flakes are still present here and there but they should be forcefully peeled out. Now a thorough saline lavage has to be given to dilute and wash out any remaining traces of infected fluid. The abdomen will be closed with a drain placed in pouch of Douglas.

Delayed Primary Closure
(Fig. 8.26a–c)

This wound is of a patient who underwent laparotomy for pelvic abscess (Fig. 8.26a). She had undergone LSCS elsewhere a few days earlier and was referred to us with high-grade fever. Laparotomy was done through a vertical incision, and this explains why the patient now has an inverted T-shaped wound. The rectus sheath has been closed, and the skin was not closed. One can see that there are no suture marks on the skin, and the suture knots on the rectus sheath are intact.

Daily dressing was done with povidone iodine pack till health granulation tissue appeared all around and the patient came out of sepsis. This image is of the wound on day 2 of laparotomy. One can see that the subcutaneous fat is pale and poorly vascularized. The wound would surely have gaped had the skin been closed at the time of laparotomy.

The same wound after a week (Fig. 8.26b). Healthy granulation tissue has started forming,

Fig. 8.25

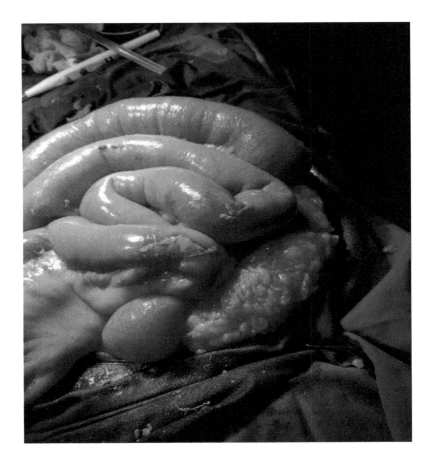

Fig. 8.26a

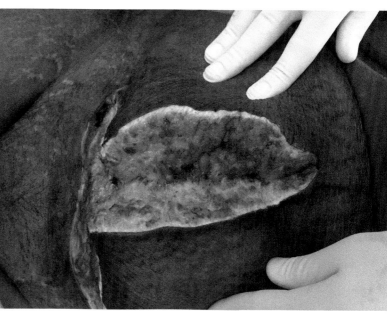

Fig. 8.26b

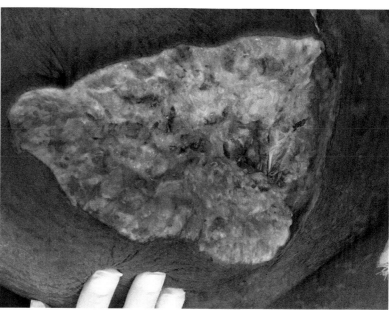

but there is still a lot of slough. One can see that nonabsorbable suture has been used for closure of rectus and that there is a defect in the rectus sheath. The peritoneum however is intact. This is the advantage of a layered suture in cases of vertical incision. Should the rectus sheath sutures give way, the sutured peritoneum holds the abdominal contents and prevents evisceration. But then, one has to control postoperative problems like cough, vomiting, and straining due

to constipation. Sutures will give way irrespective of the type of closure if there is significantly raised intra-abdominal pressure.

The same wound is now healthy and ready for closure (Fig. 8.26c). There is pink healthy granulation tissue all over. Anemia has been corrected, and the patient is out of sepsis. The wound is sure to heal well. This is DELAYED PRIMARY CLOSURE—closure of rectus sheath and deferring the skin closure by a week or so, till

Fig. 8.26c

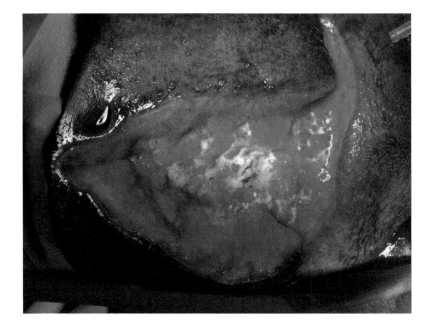

the risk factors for wound gape are corrected and controlled. Daily dressing of the wound should be done till healthy granulation tissues form all over. This greatly reduces chances of wound gape, duration of hospital stay, and treatment costs. The patient can be sent home a day after closure, and she can come for drain removal and suture removal at regular intervals. However, the risk of incisional hernia does not reduce.

It may also be advisable to close all large vertical incisions (even if they are clean contaminated wounds) by delayed primary closure, if the patient is obese and has one or more of the following risk factors—diabetes mellitus, hypoproteinemia, liver disease, previous history of radiation to abdomen, and recent chemotherapy. Adipose tissue is a poorly vascularized tissue, and obesity is a very important risk factor for wound dehiscence and burst abdomen. Wound healing is poor even in well-controlled diabetics due to defective angiogenesis and vasculopathy. Previous radiation can cause radiation-induced fibrosis and defective angiogenesis. Recent chemotherapy also has a negative impact on wound healing due to coagulation defects and defective angiogenesis. Therefore, primary closure of a vertical incision in an obese patient carries a high risk for dehiscence even if it is clean contaminated wound [9–11].

References

1. Mitchell C, Prabhu M. Pelvic inflammatory disease: current concepts in pathogenesis, diagnosis and treatment. Infect Dis Clin N Am. 2013;27(4):793–809.
2. Chappel CA, Weisenfeld HC. Pathogenesis, diagnosis, and management of severe pelvic inflammatory disease and tuboovarian abscess. Clin Obstet Gynecol. 2012;55(4):893–903.
3. Aimakhu CO, Olayemi O, Odukogbe AA. Surgical management of pelvic abscess: laparotomy versus colpotomy. J Obstet Gynaecol. 2003;23:71–2.
4. Al-Ghassab RA, Tanveer S, Al-Lababidi NH, Zakaria HM, Al-Mulhim AA. Adhesive small bowel obstruction due to pelvic inflammatory disease: a case report. Saudi J Med Med Sci. 2018;6(1):40–2.
5. Chiang RA, Chen SL, Tsai YC. Delayed primary closure versus primary closure for wound management in perforated appendicitis: a prospective randomized controlled trial. J Chin Med Assoc. 2012;75(4):156–9.
6. Verdam FJ, et al. Delayed primary closure of the septic open abdomen with a dynamic closure system. World J Surg. 2011;35(10):2348–55.
7. Deshmukh SN, Maske AN. Mass closure versus layered closure of midline laparotomy incisions: a prospective comparative study. Int Surg J. 2018;5(2):584–7.
8. Hirasawa H, Oda S, Nakamura M. Blood glucose control in patients with severe sepsis and septic shock. World J Gastroenterol. 2009;15(33):4132–6.
9. Payne WG, et al. Wound healing in patients with cancer. Eplasty. 2008;8:e9.
10. Gieringer M, Gosepath J, Naim R. Radiotherapy and wound healing: principles, management and prospects. Oncol Rep. 2011;26:299–307.
11. Guo S, DiPietro LA. Factors affecting wound healing. J Dent Res. 2010;89(3):219–29.

Vaginal Hysterectomy: *How to Accomplish*

9

Vaginal hysterectomy should be the hysterectomy of choice in patients who have a certain degree of uterovaginal descent provided there is no adnexal mass/suspicious mass/no cervical or broad ligament leiomyoma or suspected sarcoma [1, 2].

Vaginal hysterectomy may also be the hysterectomy of choice in women who are very obese and in whom laparoscopy and laparotomy are going to be very difficult and are associated with high incidence of wound infection and gape, burst abdomen, and incisional hernia. Depending on the skills of the gynecologist, vaginal hysterectomy along with the removal of fallopian tubes and ovaries can be accomplished in women with an undescended uterus (non-descent vaginal hysterectomy) and also in women with the history of one or more caesarean delivery. The size of the uterus per se should not be a contraindication [1, 2]. Presence of the conditions already mentioned, namely presence of adnexal mass, broad ligament leiomyoma, cervical leiomyoma, and possibility of the leiomyoma being a sarcoma, should be a contraindication for vaginal hysterectomy. Laparoscopy should be the surgery of choice in such situations. However, one must keep in mind that even during laparoscopy and laparotomy, one should desist from using a myoma screw or morcellating the uterus, and must avoid intraoperative spillage of the tumor contents in order to avoid upstaging of a possible malignant condition. *However, this rule does not apply to advanced carcinoma of the ovary with metastatic deposits, since the question of upstaging due to intraoperative spillage does not arise. The condition is already advanced.*

While doing vaginal hysterectomy in a patient with uterovaginal descent, one must begin by sounding the bladder after emptying it in order to determine the extent of bladder. Bigger the prolapse, lower one can expect the bladder to be (large cystocele). In procidentia, one can expect the bladder to be present just above the cervix. Determining the extent of bladder by using tactile sensation of the gloved finger or by visual assessment of what appears to be the lower limit of the bladder is subjective. Sometimes in cases of very large procidentia, the entire bladder and even the parts of the ureters just above the trigone can be in the prolapsed mass (when the cervix is held with a vulsellum and pulled with moderate traction). It is always better to sound the uterus and determine the extent of the bladder and then take the incision a few millimeters below it in order to avoid bladder injury. One must remember that if the bladder injury is on the posterior wall involving the trigone, one cannot just suture the bladder rent vaginally. The ureteric orifices can get kinked and end up very close to each other, causing narrowing of the ureteric orifices, and sometimes the ureteric orifice(s) may also get included in the sutures! Injuries of this kind will require a urologist, and the repair will have to be accomplished by placing a stent in the ureter brought out per urethra. In short it will require an extensive repair [3].

© Springer Nature Singapore Pte Ltd. 2020
A. R. Podder, J. G Seshadri, *Atlas of Difficult Gynecological Surgery*,
https://doi.org/10.1007/978-981-13-8173-7_9

For the same reasons, if hysterectomy is planned following conization of the cervix, it is better to do a laparoscopic or an open hysterectomy. The extent of bladder may be just above the stump of the cervix.

After infiltrating the mucosa over the cervix with saline, take a circumferential incision over the cervix. Adrenaline can also be added to the saline infiltration, since adrenaline causes vaso-constriction and helps reduce the intraoperative bleeding. But bleeding can take place much later when the effect of adrenaline has worn off. It need not be apparent during the surgery. Adrenaline should be used cautiously in cardiac patients, and the anesthetist should be informed prior to infiltration.

The successful opening of the anterior and posterior pouches is the first major step that needs to be accomplished while doing a vaginal hysterectomy. Once the specimen is delivered out after the pouches are opened, the possibility of ureteric injury is negligible since the ureters are retroperitoneal structures, and cannot possibly be outside along the specimen. So the opening of the pouches has to be done early in the course of the surgery.

One can use dry gauze and do blunt dissection, but if the posterior pouch is adherent due to previous colpotomy or infection, or if the anterior pouch is adherent due to previous caesarean delivery, then it is better to do sharp dissection. The assistant should pull the specimen with moderate traction, while the operating gynecologist holds the vaginal mucosa held with Allis forceps with one hand and does the sharp dissection with the other. After the posterior pouch is opened, excise the posterior peritoneum along the posterior uterine wall. This facilitates descent in a case of non-descent vaginal hysterectomy. It is easier to open the posterior pouch first, and after it has been opened, the operating gynecologist can insert his nondominant hand into the pouch of Douglas and hook the uterine fundus with

fingers and separate the uterovesical fold over the prominence of his fingers. The assistant gives moderate traction to the specimen if required. However, it is not possible to hook one's fingers over the fundus after opening the posterior pouch in cases of undescended uteri especially when the specimen is very big. In such cases one has to open the anterior pouch either by blunt dissection- if the planes are well made out, or by sharp dissection- if the planes are not well made out. If there has been a previous caesarean delivery, one is justified in fearing that the bladder may be fused to the isthmus and is more likely to get injured. One can in such situations proceed with sharp dissection, pausing at every step to drain the urine and check if the urine is blood stained or not. If the urine is clear then one can be sure that the bladder has not been injured (yet!). Another tip for opening the anterior pouch in cases of previous caesarean delivery is that one can start the dissection a bit laterally, on either side of the cervix. This is a point where the incision of LSCS may not have been taken and the bladder may not be adherent at this point. If a lot of bleeding is encountered, one can safely cauterize the bleeding vessels on the surface of the specimen, but for bleeding vessels on the base of bladder, one has to be very careful. The bleeding vessel must be caught with a fine tip forceps and gently lifted off the bladder wall before cauterizing it, as a quick "tough and go." One must make sure that the cautery settings are appropriate before starting the surgery. A cautery burn on the bladder wall should be avoided. If there is a lot of bleeding, apply pressure and think *Am I in the right plane? Or am I going into the substance of the cervix? Why should there be so much bleeding if one is in the right plane?*

Once both the pouches are opened and the color of the urine is clear, one can safely clamp, cut, and transfix the uterosacral ligaments and then clamp, cut, and ligate the uterine arteries. The cardinal rule in hysterectomy abdominal or vaginal, is that subsequent clamps must always be applied medial to the preceding clamp. Thus, the uterine clamp should be applied medial to the uterosacral pedicle and the cornual clamp is applied medial to the uterine pedicle. In an abdominal hysterectomy, the sequence is the other way—uterine clamp is always applied medial to the cornual pedicle, and the uterosacral clamp is always applied medial to the uterine pedicle.

But what does one do when it is not possible to open the anterior pouch? In such situations, one can apply clamps on the either side of the cervix, making sure that only a small length of tissue is included. The bladder can be sounded again to check if it is really high up before proceeding to cut and transfix. Releasing the uterosacral ligaments on either side will facilitate some descent.

Fothergill's surgery, also known as Manchester repair, is a procedure indicated for uterovaginal prolapse where there is an elongation of cervix and preservation menstrual function is desired. This surgery involves amputation of the cervix followed by plication of the uterosacral ligaments in front of the cervix. Therefore, one can clamp, cut, and transfix the uterosacrals even if it is not possible to open the pouches. But in order to proceed with vaginal hysterectomy further, that is, ligation of the uterine arteries, the pouches have to be opened.

Once the uterine arteries are ligated on both sides, the vascular supply to the uterus is cut off and one can bisect or morcellate, or core out the uterus. Bisection, morcellation, or coring out of the uterus reduces the bulk of the uterine fundus and helps by facilitating descent. It also provides more space for applying clamps in case of nondescent vaginal hysterectomy. But one has to remember that the uterus also gets its blood supply from the uterine branch of ovarian arteries, and the specimen can in some cases still be vascular. There can be a lot of bleeding during bisection/coring/morcellation of the uterus if the uterine branch of ovarian artery is very big. If the uterus is very fleshy, bulky, and vascular for a postmenopausal woman, think of the possibility of sarcoma and avoid morcellation to avoid intraoperative spillage of a possible malignant condition. It is advisable to convert the surgery to a staging laparotomy. For the same reason, it is better to do a staging laparoscopy or a laparotomy and avoid using a myoma screw in those women who have a sudden increase in the size of a leiomyoma or appearance of a new leiomyoma after menopause [4].

Another special situation is atypical complex hyperplasia of the endometrium. This condition is associated with foci of carcinoma endometrium which may have been missed during endometrial sampling or D&C. Therefore, one must remove the uterus without morcellation and must cut it open after it has been removed to look for any endometrial growth and gross signs of myometrial invasion. This holds true even when the hysterectomy is being done laparoscopically or by laparotomy for complex atypical hyperplasia; one must avoid any kind of morcellation or splitting open of the uterine cavity in situ. It will result in upstaging of an early stage carcinoma endometrium. The patient and her relatives should be told about the need for restaging and completion of surgery should the histopathology report show malignancy [5].

To facilitate further descent, one can divide the round ligament and apply a stay suture on the lateral cut end. This stay suture will be of immense help should the clamps slip and the pedicle gets retracted upward and starts bleeding. By pulling the stay suture on the round ligament gently, one can hope to catch the bleeding pedicle.

Also, by splitting the round ligament a bit laterally, one can gain access to the infundibulopelvic ligament if the removal of the ipsilateral fallopian tube and ovary is desired. One can deliver the specimen out of the vagina and gently hold the ovaries and fallopian tubes with a Babcock forceps, and then clamp, cut, and transfix the infundibulopelvic ligaments. Salpingo-oophorectomy can also be done vaginally in this way.

But if it is just not possible to gain access to the infundibulopelvic ligament vaginally even after morcellating the uterus and dividing the round ligament, what can possibly be done?

No attempt must be made to pull hard, in order to bring the specimen down to clamp the infundibulopelvic ligaments. The specimen could be friable or the clamps may slip leading to profuse hemorrhage necessitating a laparotomy. One must remember that the ovarian artery is a direct branch of the descending aorta, and bleeding from a torn infundibulopelvic ligament which contains the ovarian vessels can be torrential. One option is to clamp the cornua on the ipsilateral side and remove the specimen. The salpingo-oophorectomy can be done once the uterus is out of the way. The stay suture on the round ligament can be lowered a little, and using a Babcock forceps, the fallopian tube can be held. Using a long curved clamp, one can try and hold the infundibulopelvic ligament.

Drain the bladder at intervals. This serves two purposes. First, finding clear urine assures that there has so far been no bladder or ureteric injury, and second, draining the bladder facilitates descent and makes the surgery easier. In other words, a full bladder prevents descent.

Let us now study some photographs taken during live vaginal hysterectomy. Vaginal hysterectomy for uterovaginal prolapse where the specimen is present outside the introitus, and vaginal hysterectomy of a bulky undescended uterus both can be equally challenging.

Taking an Incision Over the Cervix (Fig. 9.1a–c)

The cervix is being held with a vulsellum and is being pulled with moderate traction (Fig. 9.1a). Bladder has been emptied. The white arrow is showing the metal catheter which is being used to determine the extent of the bladder. The prominence formed by the tip of the metal catheter in the lower part of the prolapse, as shown by the black arrow, is the extent of the bladder. In case of a large prolapse, or procidentia, the extent of bladder could be just above the cervix, and if the extent is not well noted before taking the incision, the bladder injury is certain.

A circumferential incision being taken over the cervix well below the extent of bladder (Fig. 9.1b). One can infiltrate the mucosa with saline prior to taking the incision. This helps in separating the surgical planes and makes wet dissection possible, especially in cases where there is vaginal atrophy due to long-standing prolapse or menopause.

The circumferential incision is being extended all around the cervix, making sure the incision is well below the extent of the bladder (Fig. 9.1c). It is better to keep the incision low even in the posterior part of the prolapse. This will provide a greater length of vagina for vault suspension at the end of the procedure.

Fig. 9.1a

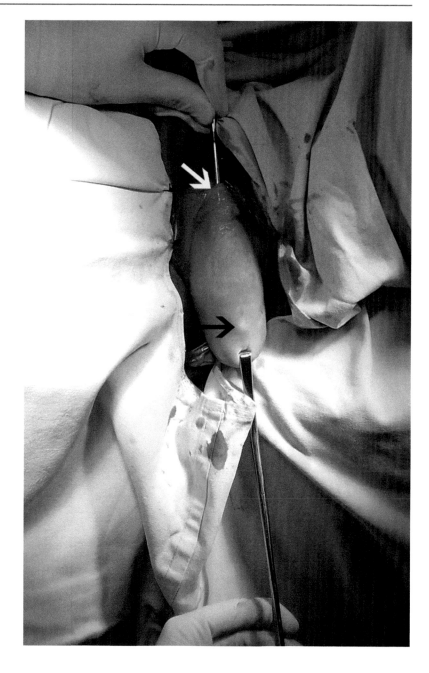

Fig. 9.1b

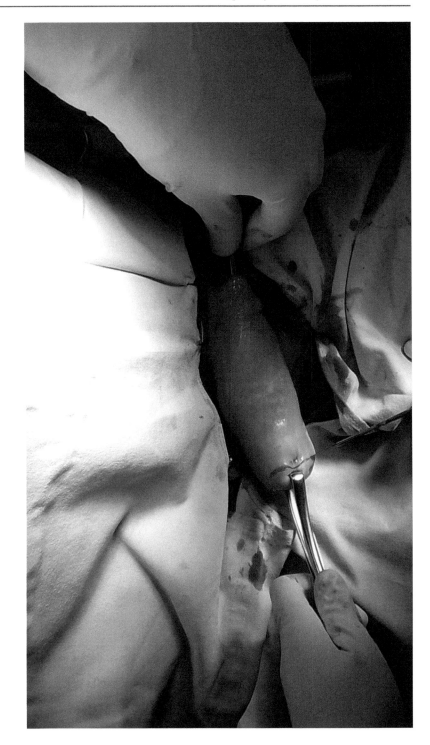

Fig. 9.1c

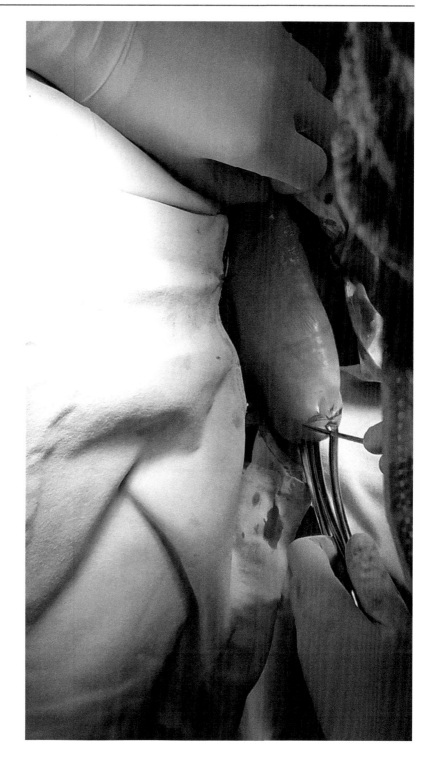

Sharp Dissection to Separate the Bladder and to Open the Anterior Pouch (Fig. 9.2a, b)

If the vaginal mucosa is moist and if there has been no previous LSCS, or previous vaginal surgery (e.g., Fothergill's repair), the bladder can easily be pushed up with dry gauze. But if for any reason this is not possible, then sharp dissection is always recommended (Fig. 9.2a). The dissection should be done staying as close to the

specimen as possible. Opening the posterior pouch first helps when the bladder is adherent as in this case.

Care has to be taken that one remains close to the specimen during sharp dissection (Fig. 9.2b).

If bleeding is noted, then the bleeding vessels should be held with a fine tip forceps or an artery forceps and cauterized. Cautery can be used safely on the specimen, but one has to be careful while using it on the base of bladder.

Fig. 9.2a

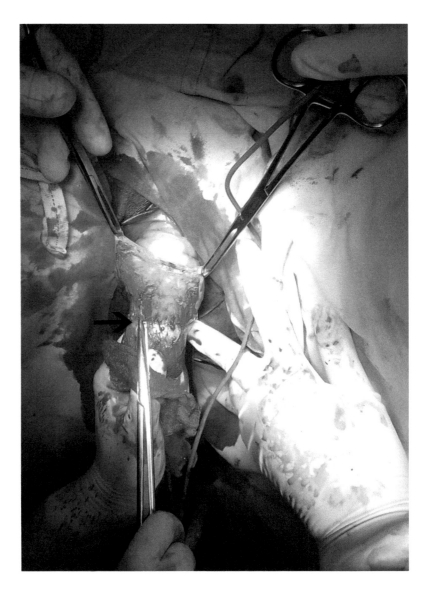

Fig. 9.2b

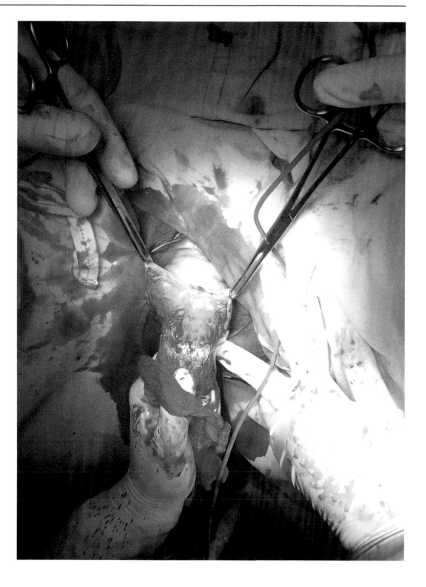

If excessive bleeding is noticed while dissecting, then one should check if one is in the correct plane. Is the dissection being done into the specimen? A few myometrial fibers left behind can theoretically grow to become a leiomyoma or a sarcoma provided there is an intact blood supply.

The author once had a patient who presented with pain in abdomen which began a few months following vaginal hysterectomy. On examination, there was a firm mass felt on the right side of the vaginal vault. The tumor markers were normal. On table there was a

6 × 6 cm leiomyoma adjacent to the right round ligament. Probably a part of myometrium in the right cornua was not fully included in the clamp and was left behind. Since the remnant continued to receive blood from the uterine branch of ovarian artery, it continued to grow and became a leiomyoma. All that was required was removal of the leiomyoma and bilateral salpingo-oophorectomy. The patient had attained menopause well before vaginal hysterectomy, and both the fallopian tubes and ovaries were vestigial organs. This case was done well before the idea for this book was conceived.

Fig. 9.3

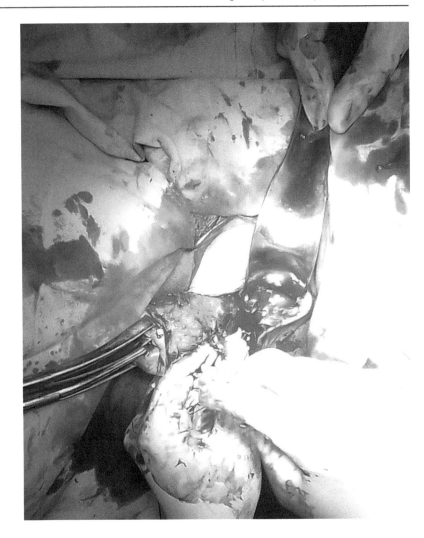

Anterior Pouch Opened (Fig. 9.3)

The anterior pouch has been opened (Fig. 9.3). One can see a clear fluid coming out through the anterior pouch; the yellow tissue is the omentum, which confirms that the anterior pouch has been opened. The gynecologist can ask for head low position if the bowels or the omentum is coming out into the operating field.

If there is gush of watery fluid and if one is not sure if the bladder has been injured, then a metal catheter can be gently inserted per urethra and the color of the urine checked. If the urine is blood stained, it is very likely that the bladder

or the ureter is injured. If one can see the tip of the catheter through an opening, then surely the bladder has been injured.

In this image, the assistant is applying pressure on a lateral bleeding vessel which needs to be identified and secured.

Clamping the Uterosacral Ligament (Fig. 9.4)

Both anterior and posterior pouches have been opened (Fig. 9.4), and a Sims speculum has been inserted into the anterior and posterior pouches.

Fig. 9.4

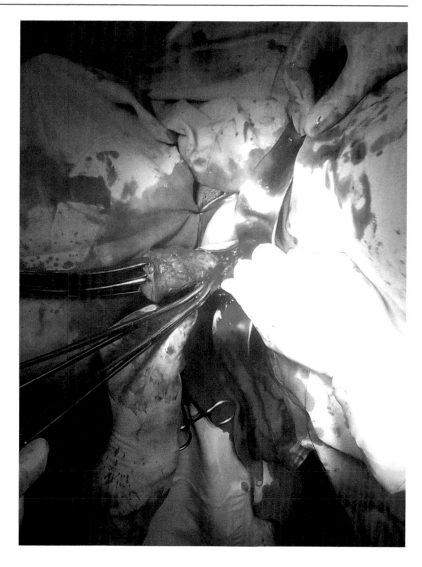

The uterosacral ligaments are now being clamped, cut, and transfixed. The clamps have been applied as close as possible to the specimen. One can appreciate the elongated cervix.

What to do when there isn't much Uterovaginal Descent? (Fig. 9.5a, b)

In Fig. 9.5a, there is not much uterovaginal descent. The posterior pouch has been opened. The operating gynecologist has held the posterior peritoneum and is stretching it. The gloved finger

is acting like a guard, so that the rectum located behind does not get injured. The arrow is showing the plane along which the peritoneal attachment can be incised.

A close-up view (Fig. 9.5b), the posterior peritoneum is being incised to facilitate greater descent. The peritoneum is being stretched with a finger. After making sure that there is no other structure between the peritoneum and the gloved finger, the peritoneum is being incised along the posterior uterine surface. By releasing the peritoneum along the posterior uterine surface, two things are achieved. First, it will facilitate

Fig. 9.5a

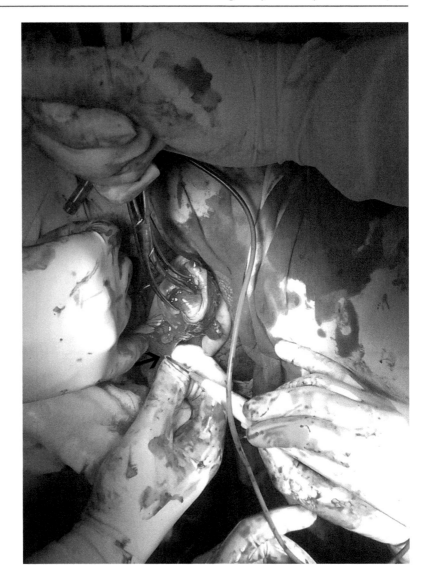

descent since the uterus is no longer held by its posterior peritoneal attachment. Second, it provides better visualization by allowing the operating gynecologist to insert a bigger speculum. The next step would be to open the anterior pouch. The operating gynecologist can insert his hand into the opened posterior pouch and hook the uterine fundus with his fingers. This will show the plane along which the dissection must be done. If the bladder is still low down, then one must separate it till it is pushed high up. Once the gloved fingers are seen through the vesico-uterine fold of the peritoneum, one can be sure that the bladder has been pushed sufficiently high up. The vesico-uterine fold can now be incised close to the specimen to open the anterior pouch. But if the uterus is very big and the operating gynecologist cannot insert his fingers and hook the fundus, then gentle sharp dissection must be done staying close to the specimen.

Fig. 9.5b

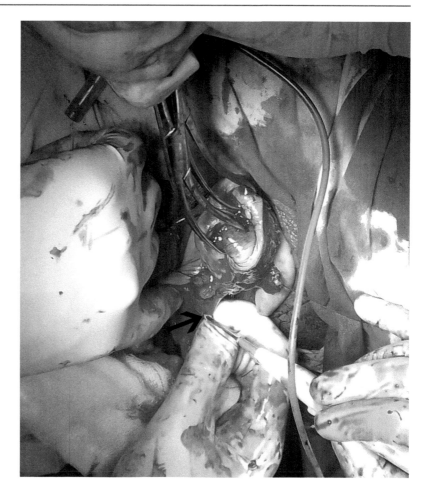

Can't Open the Anterior Pouch: What to Do? (Fig. 9.6a–c)

When it is not possible to open the anterior pouch due to an undescended uterus or due to the fact that the bladder is very high up as seen in Fig. 9.6a, one can proceed with clamping the uterosacral ligaments, provided the clamps are applied well below the bladder. One can appreciate both the uterosacrals have been clamped, cut, and transfixed, but the anterior pouch has still not been opened. There is an elongated cervix. The bladder is still high up. The arrow is showing the uterosacral stump. It is

important that the next clamp, i.e., the uterine clamp is applied medial to this stump and as close to the specimen as possible to prevent uretric injuries. But the anterior and posterior pouches should have been opened in order to proceed further, i.e., to clamp the uterines. One can clamp the uterosacral ligament before the pouches are opened if one is sure that the bladder is high up. Dividing the uterosacral ligaments will facilitate some descent, and one can attempt opening the pouches again. But it is inadvisable to clamp the uterines without the pouches being opened. Remember, the ureter is the "water under the bridge," and it runs below the uterine artery.

Fig. 9.6a

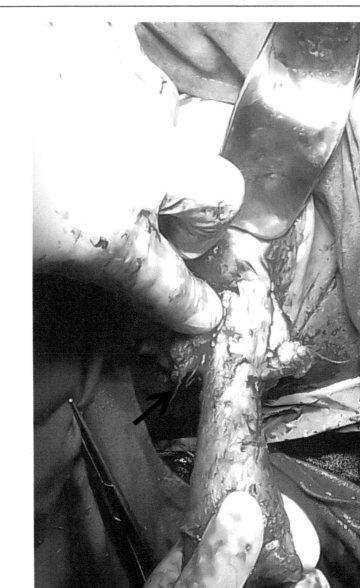

The pouches have to be opened and the specimen brought out before the clamping of the uterines is attempted, otherwise the possibility of bladder and ureteric injuries is very high.

The anterior pouch has still not been opened (Fig. 9.6b). The smooth peritoneum of the anterior uterine surface is not yet visible. Both the uterosacral ligaments have been clamped, cut, and transfixed. One can now better appreciate the elongation of the cervix and that some uterovaginal descent has resulted after the release of the uterosacral ligaments. This patient has had

Fig. 9.6b

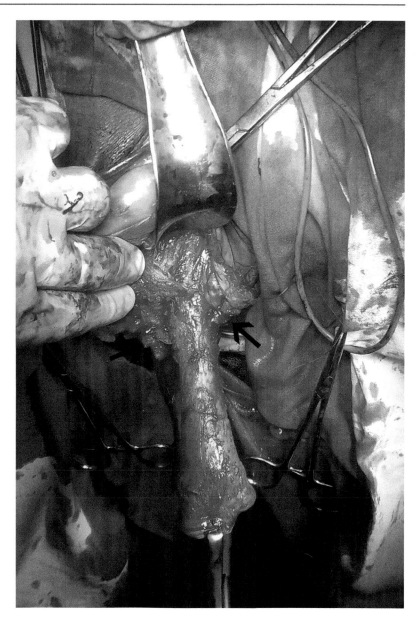

a previous cesarean delivery, and the bladder is densely adherent to the uterus. Earlier, most obstetricians believed in closing the uterovaginal fold following closing the uterine incision after delivering the baby by cesarean section.

The belief was that this step was important to

– Prevent scar endometriosis should the decidua spill into the peritoneal cavity.
– Prevent spillage of infected uterine contents, since membranes would have ruptured in most

cases and ascending infection from the vagina is possible.

This is now known not to be true. In fact, it creates the problem of an "advanced bladder"/"high up bladder" during future hysterectomy [6]. So how does one open the anterior pouch in such situations? In the above example, the plane is still not well appreciated even after considerable dissection.

The gynecologist has inserted a finger into the anterior space (Fig. 9.6c). As one can see the

Fig. 9.6c

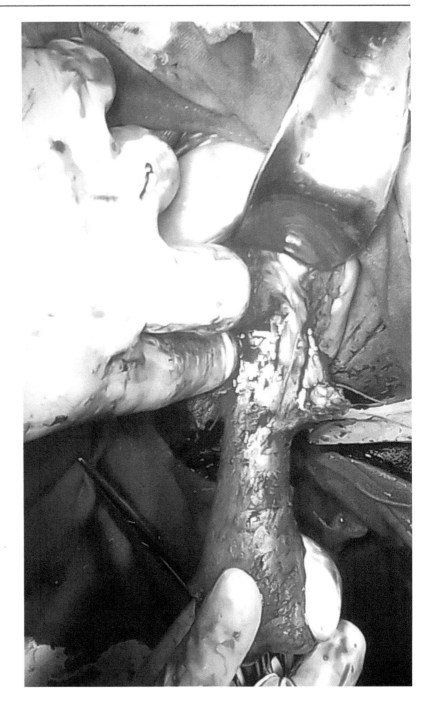

anterior pouch has been opened a bit laterally. In those cases with a history of previous caesarean delivery, one can expect difficulties in opening the anterior pouch and the bladder to be high up. A point a bit laterally on the isthmus can serve as a window where the uterovesical fold can be felt and opened. In this example, both the uterosacrals have been clamped, cut, and transfixed. One cannot proceed further without opening the anterior pouch. One must empty the bladder time to time to check the color of the urine and also to keep it empty. A full bladder hinders descent of the specimen. The patient may have received a lot of IV fluids to counter spinal hypotension. Hence, the bladder may fill fast.

Deliver the Specimen Out (Fig. 9.7)

The anterior pouch has been successfully opened, and the specimen has been delivered outside (Fig. 9.7). The huge fundus and an elongated cervix can be appreciated. With the help of a suction cannula, the assistant is helping the gynecologist locate the bleeding vessels.

Clamping the Uterines (Figs. 9.8 and 9.9a, b)

The horizontal arrow is pointing to the knuckle of the uterine artery (Fig. 9.8). It is located at the isthmus, which can be appreciated in the above image. The arrow pointing down is pointing to the friable bleeding tissue. The gynecologist has

Fig. 9.7

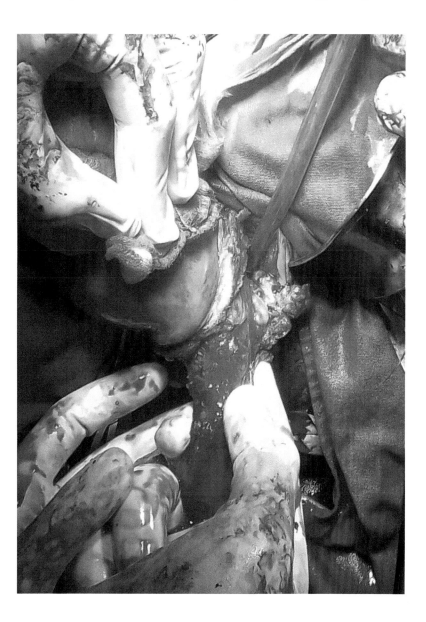

Fig. 9.8

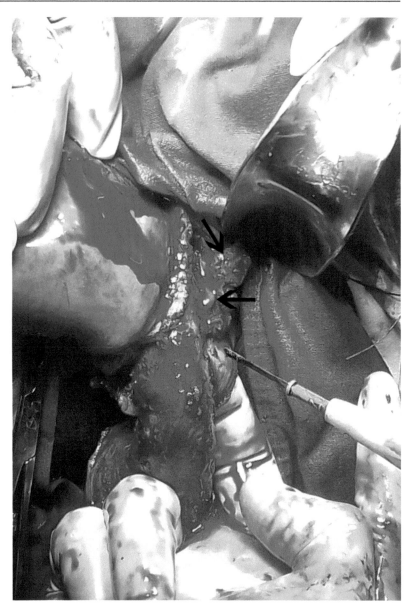

hooked the posterior peritoneum with finger and is trying to incise it. As mentioned earlier, this will release the uterus from its posterior attachment and will facilitate further descent. The uterine clamp can be applied immediately afterward. Releasing the posterior peritoneum will also provide some more space for the clamps to be applied.

One should not apply too much of traction and forcibly apply clamps (when there is little space). First, the tissue could be friable and the clamp can slip. And should the clamp holding a major vessel slip, there can be profuse bleeding. The muscle fibers in the pedicle will retract, and it will be very difficult to catch the pedicle from below. This will make laparotomy necessary. Second, it can lead to injuries; hence, applying clamps blindly is strongly discouraged. One must know what one is cutting and where one is taking a stitch. Third, it will hinder secure knotting, because there is very little space to securely place the knots. The knots may appear secure with the specimen still in situ and with the assistant giving moderate traction.

Fig. 9.9a

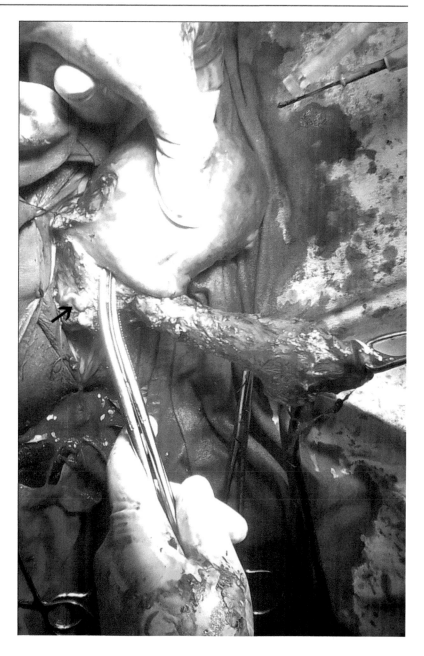

But they will become loose once the surgery is completed, and this will create problems later in the postoperative period. A hematoma/collection can form in the pouch of Douglas which can present as diarrhea and fever [7].

The uterine artery is a tortuous vessel at the level of the isthmus (Fig. 9.9a). The arrow is pointing to the right-sided uterine artery. The clamp has been applied close to the specimen and medial to the uterosacral pedicle. With the entire specimen being outside, the possibility that ureter will get included in the clamp is ruled out.

The uterine artery has been clamped (Fig. 9.9b). In this example, the specimen has been delivered outside. But in case the descent is still not sufficient to deliver the specimen out, one can either bisect the specimen as shown by the straight black line or core out the fundus. Care

Fig. 9.9b

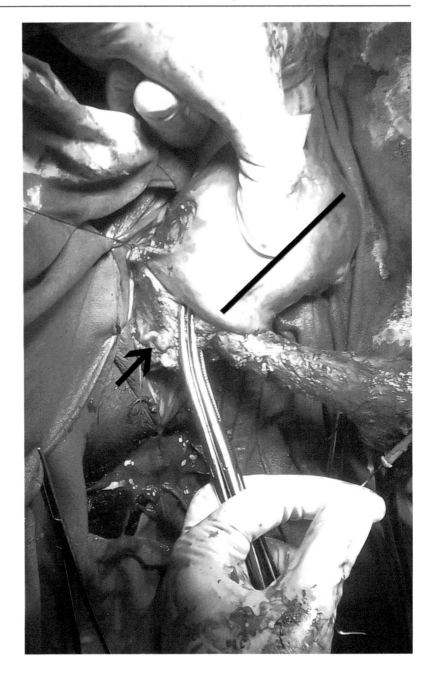

has to be taken not to injure the urethra, vaginal walls, or the bowels while bisecting/morcellating the uterus. Should the cautery electrode come in contact with the metal retractor, a large cautery burn will occur.

But one must remember that though the blood supply to the specimen has been cut off following clamping and ligation of the uterine arteries, the specimen may still be receiving a significant blood supply through the uterine branch of ovarian arteries.

In women with cervical leiomyoma and broad ligament leiomyoma, it is better to accomplish the hysterectomy by either by laparotomy or

Fig. 9.10a

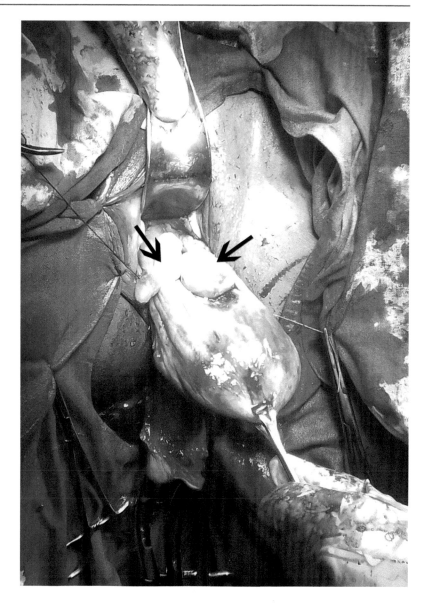

laparoscopy. And if there is a possibility that the leiomyoma is a sarcoma, the case should immediately be converted into a staging procedure. Morcellation or bisection during vaginal hysterectomy is strongly discouraged.

The same holds true while operating on a case of complex atypical hyperplasia of the endometrium. The specimen has to be removed without any kind of morcellation. Foci of carcinoma endometrium can exist which may have been missed in the preoperative evaluation.

Salpingo-Oophorectomy During Vaginal Hysterectomy (Figs. 9.10a, b and 9.11a–c)

Another trick to facilitate descent is to clamp and divide the round ligaments (Fig. 9.10a). This will also make the specimen more mobile by releasing the stabilizing force on both sides.

In Fig. 9.10a, both the ovaries and fallopian tubes have been delivered out along with the specimen. They can be removed if there is

Fig. 9.10b

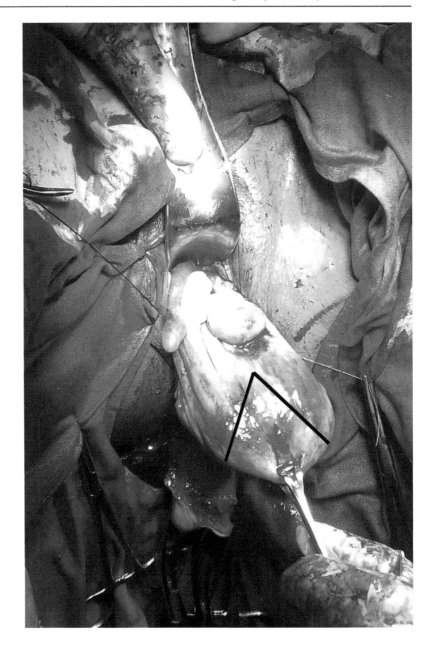

an indication, for example, in postmenopausal women where the ovaries have long ceased to function.

What can be done if the fundus cannot be delivered outside? What can be done if the cornual clamp cannot be applied, even in small installments, or even after dividing both the round ligaments?

In such situations, one can excise a wedge of the fundus as shown by the black lines (Fig. 9.10b).

This step will reduce the volume of the uterine fundus and create more space for the application of clamps. In this example, morcellation or bisection was not required since the fundus could easily be delivered outside. But if attempted, morcellation or bisection should be done below upwards. The specimen should be divided from cervic to fundus; or the myometrium should be split from isthmus to fundus along the posterior and anterior surfaces. Excessive traction can

Fig. 9.11a

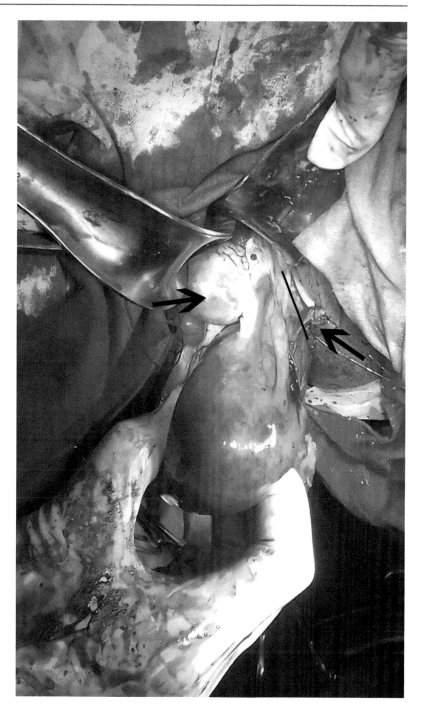

result in the cervix getting detached from the bulkier fundus, and this can result in a situation where the operating gynecologist can find it difficult holding the specimen. Excessive traction can also result in the entire specimen being "plucked out" leading to profuse hemorrhage.

Proceeding to remove the fallopian tube and ovary (Fig. 9.11a), the arrow immediately below the Sims speculum is pointing to the patient's left ovary. One can appreciate that there is a simple cyst in the ovary. The arrow pointing to the left is showing the stump of the round

Fig. 9.11b

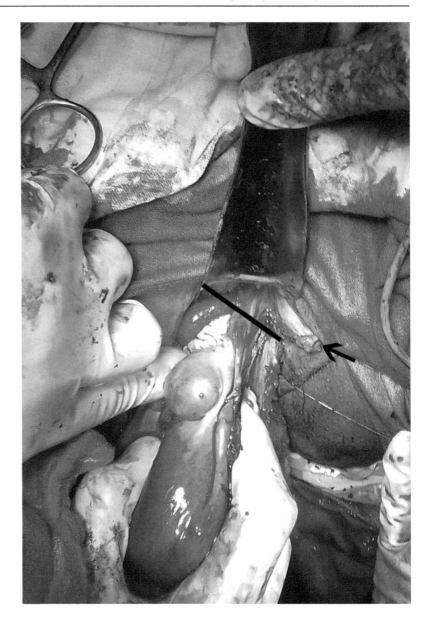

ligament which has been divided, and there is a stay suture on the lateral cut end. The black line between the cut round ligament is the plane where one can apply the clamps on the infundibulopelvic ligament.

The arrow is pointing to the lateral cut end of the round ligament (Fig. 9.11b). The space has been developed between the round ligament and the fallopian tube. Now, one can safely clamp

the infundibulopelvic ligament and remove the left ovary and the fallopian tube intact.

The infundibulopelvic ligaments have been finally clamped (Fig. 9.11c). The clamps have been applied as medial to the ovary as possible. There is a stout artery forceps which has been applied between the two clamps for additional security. One can now cut between the medial clamp and the stout artery forceps.

Fig. 9.11c

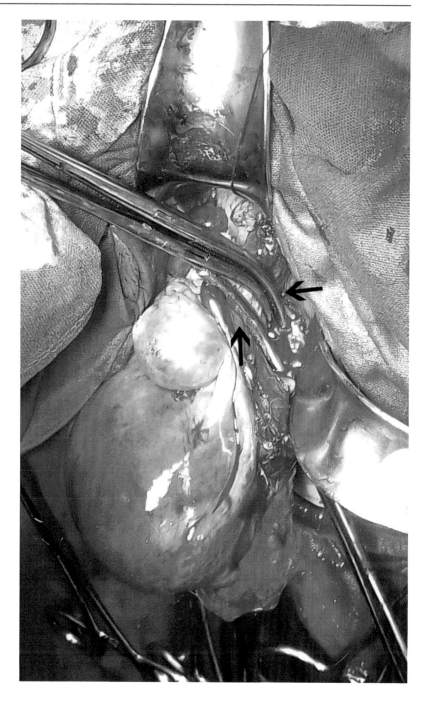

In case clamps tend to slip, that is if the clamps are not of good quality, then one can place a suture before cutting the tissue. Should the clamp slip, then one has a suture in place to hold the pedicle. The ovarian artery is a direct branch of descending aorta; should this vessel start bleeding, it will be very difficult to catch it from below. Attempts to catch it may cause further damage to the friable vessels and worsen the bleeding.

References

1. Xie QH, Liu XC, Zheng YH, Lin YJ. Indications and contraindications of vaginal hysterectomy for non-prolapsed uterus. Zhonghua Fu Chan Ke Za Zhi. 2005;40(7):441–4.
2. Balakrishnan D, Dibyajyoti G. A comparison between non-descent vaginal hysterectomy and total abdominal hysterectomy. J Clin Diagn Res. 2016;10(1):QC11–4.
3. Patil SB, Guru N, Kundargi VS, Patil BS, Patil N, Ranka K. Posthysterectomy ureteric injuries: presentation and outcome of management. Urol Ann. 2017;9(1):4–8.
4. Holzmann C, Saager C, Mechtersheimer G, Koczan D, Helmke BM, Bullerdiek J. Malignant transformation of uterine leiomyoma to myxoid leiomyosarcoma after morcellation associated with *ALK* rearrangement and loss of 14q. Oncotarget. 2018;9(45):27595–604.
5. Trimble CL, et al. Concurrent endometrial carcinoma in women with a biopsy diagnosis of atypical endometrial hyperplasia: a gynecologic oncology group study. Cancer. 2006;106:812–9.
6. Sholapurkar SL. Etiology of cesarean uterine scar defect (Niche): detailed critical analysis of hypotheses and prevention strategies and peritoneal closure debate. J Clin Med Res. 2018;10(3):166–73.
7. Farah H, et al. Postoperative pelvic pain: an imaging approach. Diagn Interv Imaging. 2015;96(10):1065–75.

Traumatic Postpartum Hemorrhage: *How to Avoid and How to Manage*

10

Traumatic PPH can occur following vaginal or caesarean delivery. Following vaginal delivery, it can occur as a result of precipitate labor, injudicious instrumental delivery, injudicious use of prostaglandins for induction of labor, injudicious use of oxytocin for augmentation of labor, malpresentations, macrosomia, and shoulder dystocia. It can occur even following a preterm vaginal delivery.

It can occur following caesarean section when the patient is taken up for caesarean section after considerable delay—when there is obstructed labor, deep transverse arrest, or when the patient is in second stage with a deeply engaged presenting part, and in cases of malpresentation when the obstetrician is unable to extract the baby without tears and extensions of the uterus.

Traumatic PPH as opposed to atonic PPH and PPH due to coagulopathy is almost always due to bad obstetric practices and lapses in judgment, unless it is a case of the patient being referred very late in the day, and there has been no further delay on the part of the attending obstetrician. Traumatic PPH is a condition that has to be prevented and rarely dealt with.

In teaching institutions, residents are taught that every primipara should be given a trial unless there is an obvious contraindication like malpresentation, placenta previa, etc., and every patient with one previous LSCS should be considered for TOLAC unless contraindicated. However, one must assess the pelvis at the onset of labor and determine if the pelvis is favorable with respect to baby size. With good uterine contractions, majority of the fetuses have good flexion and the vertex undergoes rotation. There is the "give of the pelvis" due to hormones like relaxin, because of which minor degrees of cephalopelvic disproportion can be overcome. However, what is not taken into consideration is that many women are under a lot of stress due to complications like PIH, being referred to a tertiary center in a state of emergency, and possible domestic issues. Also most Indian women have osteopenia [1]. Therefore though trail should be the norm, one must be vigilant and take findings like appearance of meconium, increasing caput, and FHR decelerations seriously.

Applying ventouse when the fetal head is still high can successfully deliver head out but can lead to shoulder dystocia. This is because the baby has been forcefully pulled down, but the head and shoulders have not undergone internal rotation [2]. Shoulder dystocia when encountered requires the obstetrician to deliver the baby by extending the episiotomy and by releasing the posterior shoulder. Thus one can expect multiple tears in the vaginal and paraurethral region and perineum.

To highlight the fact that one has a very high rate of successful vaginal deliveries, one must not create a record of having the maximum vaginal deliveries with disastrous results. Which means that the baby is in NICU for birth asphyxia and

© Springer Nature Singapore Pte Ltd. 2020
A. R. Podder, J. G Seshadri, *Atlas of Difficult Gynecological Surgery*,
https://doi.org/10.1007/978-981-13-8173-7_10

birth injuries, and the mother is having second/third/fourth-degree perineal tears with traumatic PPH, and needs multiple transfusions with prolonged ICU and hospital stay. Given such an outcome, the medical expenses are going to be huge and the baby's development might also be compromised.

When the baby's head is not coming out despite the cervix being fully dilated and good uterine contractions present, one must consider possibilities like cord around neck, true cord knot, constriction ring, occipito-posterior presentation, impending scar dehiscence in cases of previous LSCS, and CPD. One must review - *is the head truly descended or is it the caput which is increasing?* The decision to take the patient for an LSCS must be taken well in time. The mere fact that FHR is not showing significant decelerations should not be the sole criterion to continue giving a trial. Prolonged labor especially in second stage, where the mother has been bearing down for quite some time, is associated with multiple problems (e.g., risk of future prolapse), and performing an LSCS in such a patient is not always easy. The lower segment will be thinned out, the fetal presenting part could be deeply engaged, or there could be DTA. Difficulty in delivery is associated with tears extending down into the lower segment and laterally into the uterine arteries.

In case of prolonged trial in a patient with one previous LSCS, there is a risk of impending rupture, or even complete uterine rupture. The patient may have bled significantly by the time the abdomen is opened. The tissues can be very friable and can bleed wherever a bite is taken, and suturing can be very difficult. And if the membranes have been ruptured for a long time, there could be ascending infection, and very little liquor. The uterus would have gripped the baby, making delivery difficult.

Traumatic PPH following a vaginal delivery can be due to extension of episiotomy, perineal tears, paraurethral tears, vaginal lacerations, and rarely colporrhexis. When more than the usual bleeding is noted, the obstetrician must immediately put a mop in the vagina and ensure that there are two patent IV lines present. Oxytocin infusion must be started; methylergometrine

should be given IV if not contraindicated; bladder catheterized to monitor urine output—this is an indicator of organ perfusion, and call for help. Blood sample should be sent for crossmatch if not sent earlier. An assistant should continuously monitor the vitals and must reassure the patient, keeping an eye if the patient is getting drowsy or disoriented. The obstetrician must check if the placenta and membranes are fully expelled. If the placenta and membranes have not been expelled fully, then they should be removed by controlled cord traction. Clots should be removed and uterine massage be done to contract the uterus. If the bleeding is manageable, then the suturing can be done in the labor room itself, with patient being given IM sedation and local infiltration.

The author would like to point out that many seniors with years of experience are very quick and efficient. They suture a small episiotomy or a small tear in one continuous layer, sometimes before the placenta is expelled. This should not be a problem given the years of experience of some consultants. Episiotomy rarely gapes despite being subjected to constant friction and movement due to limb ambulation. Perineum is a naturally contaminated region of the human body. Despite these factors, episiotomy rarely gapes probably because of good blood supply.

However, this is not what the younger obstetricians and gynecologists should practice. One must wait for the placenta and membranes to be expelled and remove all clots and membrane remnants. The placenta needs to be examined for any missing lobe or abnormalities. One must remember that missing cotyledons can cause profuse vaginal bleeding later, and some placental abnormalities are associated with fetal anomalies [3]. If any placental abnormality is found, the neonatologist has to be informed. After suturing the episiotomy, one is reluctant to explore the vagina since one would not want to disturb the sutures. The practice of tightly packing the vagina is strongly discouraged. If the bleeding is significant and hinders good visualization, a mop must be inserted only till the patient is shifted to the OT for exploration and suturing under GA. For these reasons, it is prudent to wait till the placenta and membranes are fully expelled, the vagina is explored with good illumination before beginning to suture the episiotomy. The separation of placenta should not take more than a few minutes.

After the placenta and membranes are expelled fully and the uterus well contracted, the patient must be given lithotomy with IM sedation given, and bladder catheter in situ. The lips of the cervix should be held with two sponge holders side by side. The assistant should expose the vagina with two Sims speculums. The obstetrician can explore clockwise or counterclockwise and check for any cervical tears and colporrhexis. As the obstetrician moves from one point to another, the sponge holders are released and reapplied further along the cervix, while the assistant moves the two Sims speculums in the direction of the exploration. Any tear should be sutured taking care to go a little beyond the apex of the tear. Should there be colporrhexis or profuse bleeding which obstructs visualization, the patient must be quickly shifted to the OT for exploration and repair under GA.

After the cervical tears are sutured, one must begin suturing the episiotomy and the vaginal tears. Come from above downward. One can visualize the lower tears only after the bleeding from the upper most tear has been controlled. Care must be taken to go beyond the apex of each tear, lest the tear continues to bleed from the point above the highest stitch. If the apex cannot be visualized, then one can insert a tampon or a small mop in the vagina. This will apply pressure on the other tears and may help in locating the apex of the episiotomy/tear that is being sutured. If the apex is still not visualized, take a stitch as high as possible and apply gentle traction to the suture material. This should help is lowering and bringing out the part of the episiotomy/tear above the point of the stitch. One can then take stitches above this point. If the episiotomy is very big due to extension, sometimes the ischiorectal pad of fat is exposed, then one has to close this space with interrupted sutures after securing the apex. It will be very difficult to close the middle layer between the mucosa and the perineal skin once the entire mucosa is sutured. Unsecured bleeding vessels in this layer can result in vulval hematoma. This space can accommodate a large volume of blood. The patient can silently bleed

and can land in hypovolemic shock and severe anemia. Thus severe pain and discomfort at the episiotomy site should be checked promptly, never dismissed. There could be a huge vulval hematoma, which can deceptively look small due to tight skin sutures. It is only after the sutures are opened that a huge clot is revealed.

An obstetrician must make a liberal episiotomy, especially for preterm births (contrary to what one might think that small babies do not need so much of space. But then excessive compression of the head has to be avoided in preterm babies). When the head is on perineum and is stretching it, one may be reluctant to give a 5–8 cm long episiotomy, fearing that it may be very big! But once the baby is delivered, a big episiotomy will not appear so big! Taking a small episiotomy and then applying ventouse or forceps is another disastrous step. A single 5–8 cm long mediolateral episiotomy is easy to suture than multiple tears and lacerations caused due to delivery of a big baby through narrow birth canal as a result of a small episiotomy. If the ischiorectal pad of fat is seen, then it indicates extension of the episiotomy.

Small paraurethral tears can be left alone if there is no bleeding, but if they need to be sutured, then a per urethral catheter is a must. Not only does it help is monitoring urine output, but more importantly it prevents a stitch being taken through the urethral lumen during suturing of a paraurethral tear. The catheter has to be left in situ for a few days if a paraurethral tear is present. This is an extremely pain-sensitive area, and the patient may not feel bladder fullness when there are sutures in this area. Also it prevents the burning pain when urine drops come in contact with the sutures.

Third-degree perineal tears involving the edge of the anal sphincter can be sutured in labor room with good local infiltration provided the patient is stable and cooperative. But all fourth-degree perineal tears involving the rectum, all tears where the patient is bleeding profusely, those patients in severe pain, and hemodynamically unstable patients should be sutured in the OT under GA. It is always advisable to call a surgeon if there are rectal injuries.

In case of traumatic PPH encountered during LSCS, one has to exteriorize the uterus and quickly secure the angles of the uterine incision. If there is an extension into the uterine arteries, then one has to first secure the angle and may have to do the uterine artery ligation just below the level of the uterine incision. If there are extensions into the lower segment, then they should be sutured separately. One should not try to suture the upper and lower incisions in a straight line, since the length of the lower margin will be longer than the length of the upper margin of the incision. The thickness of myometrium at the upper and lower margins of the incision will also be different. The thickness of the upper margin will be more than that of the lower margin. The myometrium of the lower segment may be very much thinned out and the tissue integrity poor. The tissue may cut through and can bleed wherever a bite is taken. It may require very gentle suturing, and the sutures should not be tightened by pulling. Instead a mop should be used to gently pull the suture material against the tissue to tighten it.

There could be tears or extensions which could be intentional, like an inverted T incision, or a J-shaped incision, taken to deliver a baby in transverse lie, or with deeply engaged head. Even in such a scenario, each angle has to be secured separately and sutured. No attempt should be made to suture the entire length in a straight line.

If there are tears which have extended deep down or laterally, one must trace the ureters to rule out the possibility of a stitch being taken through it. One must look transperitoneally through the pouch of Douglas and locate the ureters, and check if the stitches are well above the level of the ureters. It would be advisable to call the urologist if ureteric and bladder injuries are suspected/found. Bladder injuries in a case of obstructed labor and those due to prolonged trial in a case of previous LSCS may involve the trigone or the posterior wall of bladder. It may require ureteric stenting and an extensive repair. Only a small rent in the dome of bladder can be sutured by the obstetrician [4, 5].

A Pfannenstiel incision for an LSCS for a patient in second stage is perfectly fine, even if there are other problems like uterine rupture. Even if internal iliac artery ligation becomes nec-essary, one can convert the incision to a Maylard incision and ask the anesthetist for GA.

The decision to go for internal iliac artery ligation and/or obstetric hysterectomy should never be deferred till it is too late to save the patient. It is better to operate when the patient is still stable, than when in a state of DIC and irreversible shock due to profuse hemorrhage.

Lastly, all patients who have delivered by an LSCS done in second stage of labor are poor candidates for TOLAC, and one must not subject them to a trail in next pregnancy just for sake of following a protocol. Those with tears, extensions, inverted T-shaped and J-shaped scars are not to be subjected to labor in subsequent pregnancies, even if it is a case of preterm labor or a case of IUD. They have to be taken up for elective repeat LSCS. The risks of uterine rupture are far too high.

Also, those patients who have suffered a third- or fourth-degree perineal tear in a previous pregnancy should be taken for elective repeat LSCS, though the perineal trauma could have been due to bad judgment and vaginal delivery in the present pregnancy might be safe.

Let us now study some photographs taken when traumatic PPH was encountered following vaginal delivery followed by photographs taken when traumatic PPH was encountered during LSCS.

Traumatic PPH following Vaginal Delivery (Figs. 10.1, 10.2a–c, 10.3a, b, 10.4, 10.5a–c, and 10.6)

Badly Sutured Episiotomy

An example of a badly sutured episiotomy (Fig. 10.1), it can be quite tempting to suture a small episiotomy or a perineal/vaginal tear in a single layer by taking continuous running sutures. This should not be a problem if the tear is really small. But then this is not really the method that should be followed. The mucosal layer, followed by the muscle layer and finally the skin should be sutured separately. This allows for the episiotomy/tear to be sutured in

Fig. 10.1 Badly sutured episiotomy

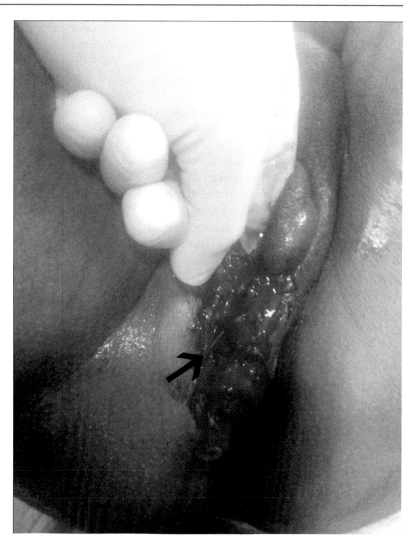

correct alignment, and it makes the obstetrician good at suturing and taking knots quickly. Following vaginal delivery, the patient is tired and is not completely still while the episiotomy/tear is being sutured. The pain relief due to local anesthesia is not 100%. When a resident practices layered closure in such situations, the resident is bound to become very quick and efficient in suturing and applying knots.

There are clots in the episiotomy incision (Fig. 10.1). The patient was complaining of severe pain at the episiotomy site. The sutures have been opened. The arrow is pointing at a catgut remnant. On close inspection of the skin edges, the suture bite marks can be appreciated along the skin margins. At the upper end of the episiotomy, there is a swelling, and the finger is inserted into the vagina, inside that part of the episiotomy where the mucosa has not been sutured. This is because of the tearing hurry on part of the obstetrician. It is now advisable to remove all sutures and close the episiotomy in layers with the patient in lithotomy position, and with careful inspection of the entire vagina under good illumination. The patient will require IM sedation, and repeat local infiltration prior to suturing.

Fortunately, the condition is discovered before a large vulval hematoma was formed.

Suturing Cervical Tears
(Fig. 10.2a–c)

Figure 10.2a shows the anterior and posterior lip of the cervix being held by sponge holders. The assistant has inserted a Sims speculum in the 11 o'clock and the 6 o'clock positions. There are two cervical tears as shown by the two straight arrows. The assistant should rotate the two Sims speculums either clockwise or counter clockwise as shown by the curved arrows, so that the obstetrician can inspect the entire cervix and vagina all around. Each tear should be sutured. Should there be profuse bleeding, multiple tears, or if the patient is in severe pain, suturing should be done in the OT under GA. If the tears are just one or two and if the patient is not bleeding heavily and is cooperative, then the suturing can be done

in the labor room under IM sedation and local infiltration.

Just adjacent to the upper Sims speculum, there is a mediolateral episiotomy, which will be sutured after suturing all the cervical, paraurethral, and vaginal tears.

A bleeding cervical tear (Fig. 10.2b), the arrow is pointing at the apex where a catgut stitch has been taken. The lips of the cervix have been held by sponge holders. Now the tear must be sutured with interlocking sutures.

A well-sutured cervical tear (Fig. 10.2c); the first suture has been taken well above the apex. The patient was hemodynamically stable, alert, and conscious. Therefore, Foley catheter has not been inserted in situ. The bladder was drained with a simple rubber catheter during second stage of labor.

Fig. 10.2a

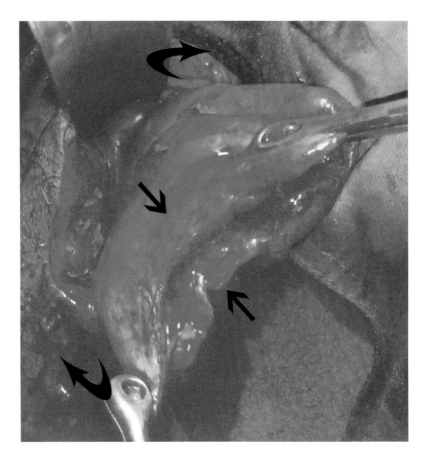

Fig. 10.2b

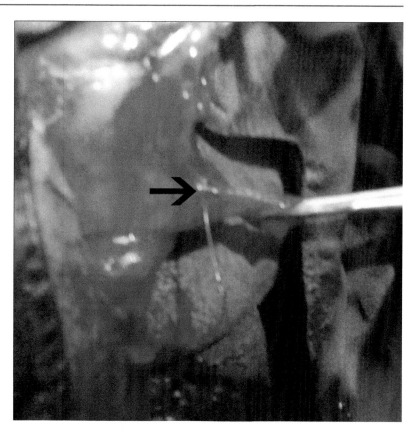

Fig. 10.2c

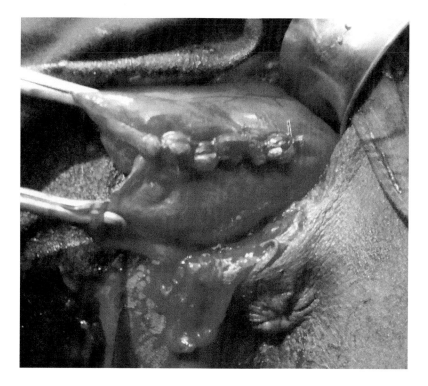

Fig. 10.3a

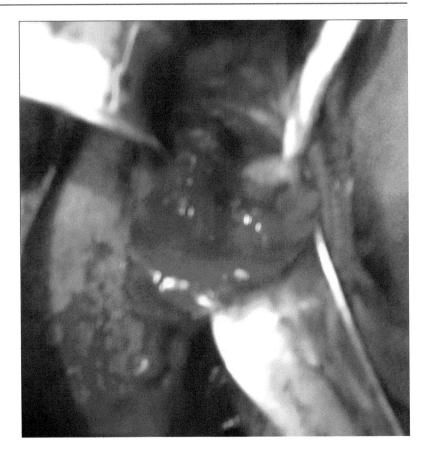

A Deep Episiotomy (Fig. 10.3a, 10.3b, 10.4, 10.5a, 10.5b, 10.5c, 10.6)

The episiotomy incision has got extended high up (Fig. 10.3a). It is better to take a liberal episiotomy than try to deliver the baby through a small episiotomy with excessive traction. When the fetal head is on perineum, there is stretching of the perineum, and the episiotomy incision may appear unduly large. But after delivery, the episiotomy will not be that big. If the baby cannot be delivered despite a liberal episiotomy of 5–8 cm, then one must empty the bladder if it has not yet been done. And if the baby still cannot be delivered, then one must seriously reconsider if vaginal delivery is possible. There could be (multiple) loops of cord around neck (very common), true knot (rare), constriction ring, or certain degree of CPD. One must also check is it the head which has descended or is it the caput? Has the head rotated? Is it occipitoposterior position?

Applying forceps or ventouse will only cause more trauma and bleeding in the mother and serious birth injuries in the baby, which could be permanent.

In Fig. 10.3a, a small mop has been inserted into the vagina to help locate the apex. The apex has still not been located.

The obstetrician must not forget to remove the vaginal mop/tampon after finishing the suturing. Care must be taken while suturing not to include a part of the mop/tampon in the stitches. The sutures will have to be removed to facilitate removal of the mop/tampon if the sutures have been taken through the mop/tampon. Remember that the patient may have had a long painful labor and has been in dorsal/lithotomy position for considerable time. She may be having leg cramps, and subjecting her endless suturing, continued pain and blood loss is deplorable.

A bleeding episiotomy where the apex has still not been identified (Fig. 10.3b). A bigger mop has

Fig. 10.3b

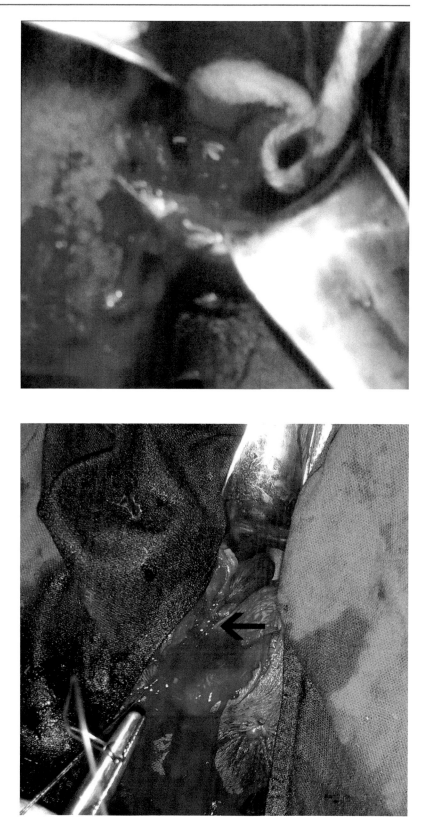

Fig. 10.4

been inserted into the vagina. Should bleeding be profuse and the patient beginning to deteriorate, then a mop must be quickly inserted and the patient shifted to the OT for suturing under GA.

When the apex of the episiotomy or a tear cannot be identified, is it always necessary to shift the patient to OT (if the patient is very much stable)?

Well, one can take a stitch as high up as possible (Fig. 10.4). The arrow is pointing to the point where a high stitch has been taken, and this suture is like a stay suture. The suture material is gently pulled down, and this will expose the part of the episiotomy/tear above the stay suture. The obstetrician can then take a bite above the stay suture well above the apex.

In Fig. 10.4, there is no bleeding above the stay suture. All the bleeding is from the episiotomy below the stay suture.

The vaginal mucosa of the episiotomy incision has been sutured (Fig. 10.5a). A sponge holder has been gently inserted into the muscle layer to show how deep the incision is. The bleeding is also significant. Closing the skin with deep mattress sutures may not suffice. If this layer is not closed with interrupted sutures, a vulval hema-

toma is likely to form. This layer can accommodate more than a liter of blood. The patient can slide into decompensated shock if the hematoma is not quickly identified, evacuated and blood loss corrected promptly with transfusions. A vulval hematoma is very painful, and severe pain at episiotomy site should be taken seriously.

An episiotomy with vaginal mucosa and muscle layer sutured (Fig. 10.5b). There is now no bleeding from the episiotomy or from the uterus. Only the skin remains to be sutured. Mattress sutures can be taken in a matter of minutes. One can appreciate the consequences if this episiotomy was sutured in a continuous running fashion from the apex to the skin!

A well-sutured episiotomy: a layered closure (Fig. 10.5c), as opposed to the one shown in Fig. 10.1.

A Huge Vaginal Hematoma (Fig. 10.6)

Another cause for obstetric trauma is the incorrect and injudicious application of forceps and ventouse. The cervix should be fully dilated, presentation must be vertex and low down,

Fig. 10.5a

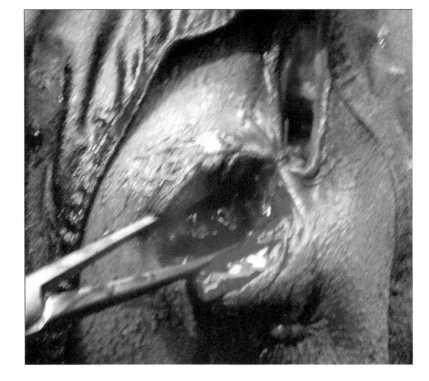

Fig. 10.5b

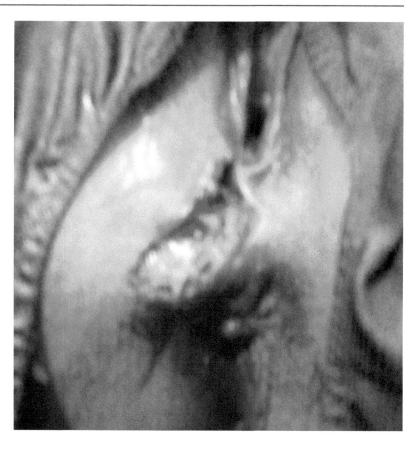

Fig. 10.5c

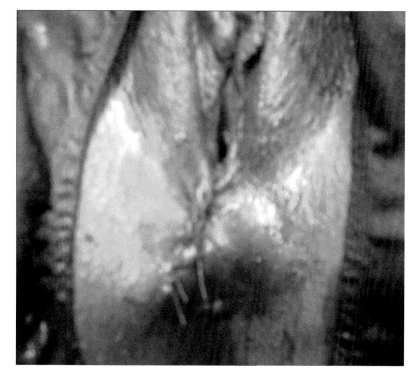

Fig. 10.6

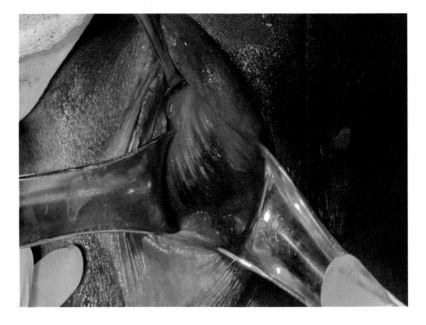

membranes ruptured, head rotated within 45°, and cephalopelvic disproportion ruled out. The obstetrician must check if the criteria for outlet forceps or low forceps application have been correctly fulfilled before inserting the forceps blades or the vacuum cup. The application technique of forceps or ventouse is not discussed here. But one highly avoidable mistake is to switch from forceps to ventouse or vice versa or repeatedly trying for instrumental delivery despite one or two pulls with moderate traction not being successful.

This patient was delivered by vacuum, and probably a fold of the vaginal wall got included between the vertex and the cup. The patient's hemoglobin dropped from 12 g% on admission to labor ward to 6 g% the day following delivery. On examination, a huge vaginal hematoma was discovered. It was drained, and bleeding vessels were secured under GA. The reason why the attending obstetrician was reluctant to perform an LSCS was that the patient had severe PIH and had come in second stage of labor. It is always better to perform an LSCS than have successful vaginal deliveries with disastrous results.

Traumatic PPH during LSCS
(Figs. 10.7a–c, 10.8a, b, 10.9a, b, 10.10, 10.11a–c, 10.12a–c, and 10.13)

Suturing when Tissues are Thinned Out and Friable (Fig. 10.7a–c)

How does one suture the uterus during LSCS when the lower segment is very much thinned out (Fig. 10.7a)? Let us say when the LSCS is being done after a prolonged trial when the tissues are friable and cuts through. In addition, the tissue bleeds wherever a bite is taken, trying to secure bleeding ends up causing more bleeding!

Well, it is better to prevent such a situation by taking up the patient for a timely LSCS. One can appreciate that the tissue integrity near the uterine angle above the Doyen's retractor is poor (Fig. 10.7a).

One must never pull the suture to tighten it (Fig. 10.7b). The obstetrician is placing the suture with the help of the needle holder. Both the angles have already been secured to begin with. One can see that there is significant bleeding from below the suture line in the midpoint.

Fig. 10.7a

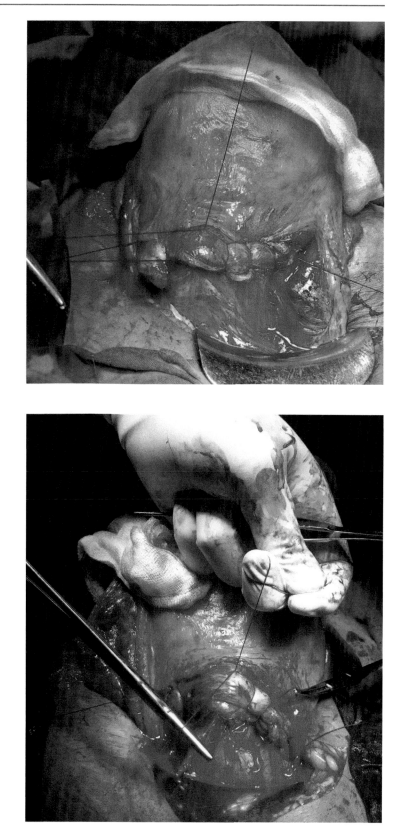

Fig. 10.7b

Fig. 10.7c

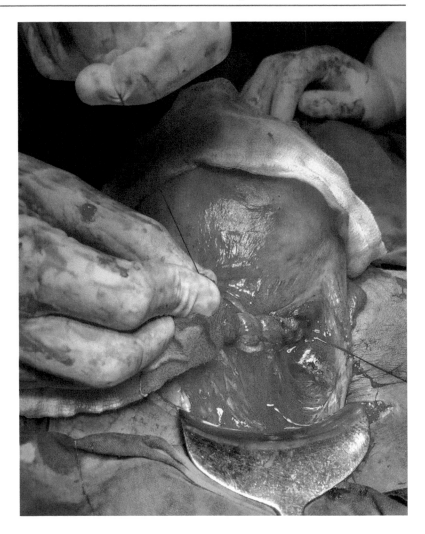

This will have to be secured by figure of eight sutures after the uterine incision is closed.

After placing the suture, the obstetrician or the assistant gently tightens the suture with the help of a mop (Fig. 10.7c). The suture is being pulled gently with a mop being used to provide counter pressure. If one just pulls the suture, then it is sure to cut through the tissues making suturing even more difficult.

Suturing a Lateral Extension
(Fig. 10.8a, b)

The angle has extended laterally into the uterine artery (Fig. 10.8a). No attempt to blindly suture should be made. The angle has to be located, and a stitch should be taken lateral to it. The arrow is pointing to the site where the angle could be located. Profuse bleeding has obscured the operating field.

The bleeding angle has been located and secured (Fig. 10.8b). The assistant must lift the fundus and help in exposing the bleeding vessel. In the above image, one can see that the angle has extended into the posterior surface of the uterus. The varying thickness of the myometrium of the upper and lower margins—the thinned out lower segment and a relatively thick upper segment—can be appreciated.

The gap in the broad ligament has to be closed lest a loop of bowel herniates and results in an internal hernia.

Fig. 10.8a

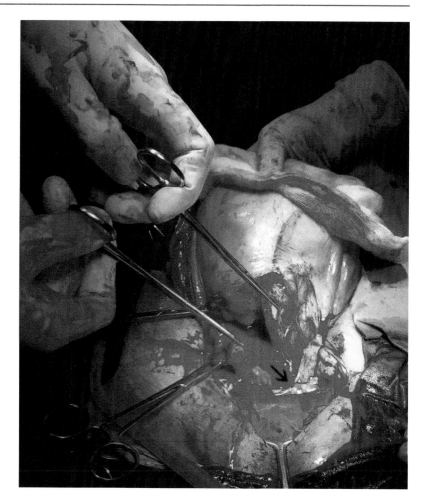

Checking the Ureter (Figs. 10.9a, b and 10.10)

After the uterus has been closed and the hemostasis secured, it is always advisable to check if the ureters are safe (Fig. 10.9a). This has to be done if there are downward or lateral extensions in the lower uterine segment. The urine is very often blood tinged due to prolonged pressure on the bladder due to prolonged trail, deep transverse arrest, etc. This does not mean that bladder or ureteric injuries have occurred. But if there have been extensions, then one must check for any possible injuries, which might have occurred as a result of sutures.

The fundus is held anteriorly by the assistant and the pouch of Douglas exposed (Fig. 10.9a). All the collected blood and amniotic fluid is suctioned out. One can see the ureters and the iliac vessels transperitoneally on the either side of the rectum. The arrow pointing down is showing the ureters seen transperitoneally. The horizontal arrow is showing a dimple. This dimple is the point where a deep stitch was taken to secure the uterine artery into which the uterine incision had extended. As one can see, the stitch appears well above the possible location of the ipsilateral ureter.

While taking a deep stitch, it is always better to exteriorize the uterus. The author always exte-

Fig. 10.8b

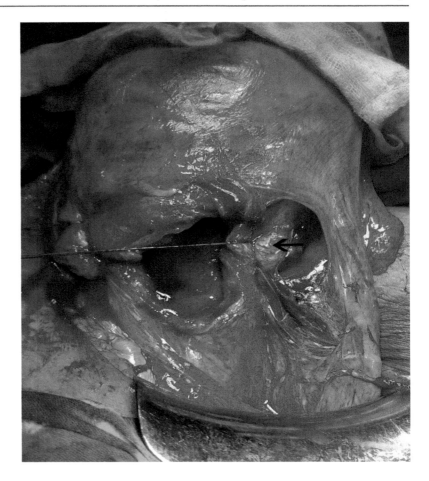

riorizes the uterus in all cases as a rule. While taking a deep stitch, one hand must be placed behind the uterus, so that the obstetrician can judge the depth of the stitch. This also prevents the uterus being stitched to the skin or the abdominal wall which are present behind when the uterus is exteriorized. If the stitch is taken with uterus in situ, then the stitch might be taken through the sigmoid or the rectum which are located behind the uterus in the pelvis.

A close-up view of the pouch of Douglas (Fig. 10.9b), the location of the ureters with respect to the deep stitch can be appreciated. The dimple as shown by the arrow pointing to the right is the point where the deep stitch was taken. The arrow pointing down is showing the contralateral ureter which is seen transperitoneally. The ipsilateral ureter is also located at the same level, and now one can be sure that

the lowest stitch and the ureter are quite far apart.

Another example: checking if the deep stitches have injured the ureter (Fig. 10.10).

The uterus has been closed after delivering the baby. There was a lateral extension of the uterine angle into the uterine artery which was secured. The uterus has been exteriorized, and the assistant is holding the fundus with slight upward traction. The pouch of Douglas has been cleared of all collected blood and fluid.

The arrow pointing down is where the ureter is located. The arrow pointing up is showing a dimple where a deep stitch has been taken to control the bleeding. A small hematoma has formed around it can be appreciated. Fortunately, it is not expanding. There is a large distance between the stitch and the ureter. So the possibility of ureteric injury is ruled out.

Fig. 10.9a

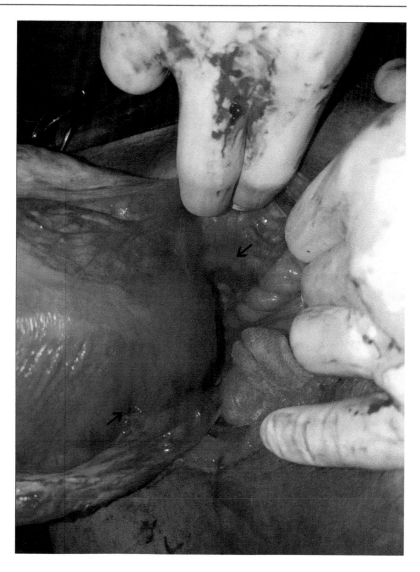

Broad Ligament Hematoma
(Fig. 10.11a–c)

A hematoma has suddenly formed during LSCS, and it is rapidly expanding in size! (Fig. 10.11a).

This is a case of primigravida with non-progress of labor. The cause was probably due to thinned out lower segment. One of the engorged vessels may have got traumatized due to retractor jerk. The bleeding point will have to be quickly located and ligated. The uterus has been exteriorized. If one attempts to control the bleeding by taking blind sutures with the uterus in situ, then one might end up taking a deep stitch through one of the posterior structures like the sigmoid on the left. If the bleeding vessel is very down below, the ureter may lie very close and may get included in the stitch.

The sutures of both the angles of the uterine incision have been kept long and are being held with artery forceps.

The uterovesical fold has been opened further and the bleeding vessel, it appears, is located somewhere down, as shown by the arrow (Fig. 10.11b). The bleeding vessels now need to be located and secured. However, one should not disturb a stable clot.

Fig. 10.9b

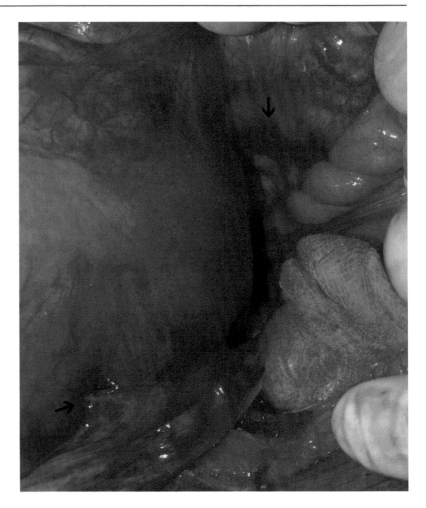

Both the uterine incision angles are well secured and the sutures have been kept long. They have been held by artery forceps (not seen in this image). As one can see, there is no bleeding from the uterine incision.

Now, if one takes blind sutures near the bleeding vessel, one can end up taking a bite through the skin or the abdominal wall if the stitch is taken with the uterus exteriorized. Or one might end up taking a stitch through the sigmoid or rectum if the stitch is taken with the uterus in situ.

So, it is advisable to first exteriorize the uterus and then hold the posterior surface with one's left hand (in case of a right-handed obstetrician) and take the stitch with the right hand.

Thus, one can judge the depth of the stitch. One should not take a good deep stitch and tightly secure it only to discover that another structure has been included behind. If the bowel or the ureter has been included, the consequences will be serious. The stitch will immediately have to be removed which might result in bleeding, controlling which can be even more difficult since the tissues around the bleeding site would have become friable.

The arrow is pointing at the broad ligament hematoma (Fig. 10.11c). This is a case of previous LSCS who was considered for TOLAC. An indiscriminately long trail was given, and when the patient was taken up for LSCS, a hematoma

Fig. 10.10

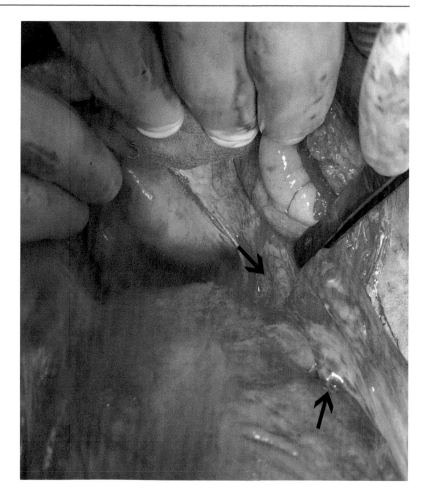

was found in the broad ligament. The uterus has been closed following delivery of the baby by LSCS. The round ligament has been cut, and the hematoma is being evacuated.

While considering a case of one previous LSCS for VBAC, one has to keep in mind the following:

– Was the previous caesarean truly an LSCS? Or is it a case of inverted T scar or J scar? Was there an extension into the uterines or any downward extension? Should a patient with unknown scar be considered for TOLAC?
– Classical signs of impending scar dehiscence are not always present, silent scar dehiscence is more common than thought. If the presenting part is persistently high despite good contractions, or if meconium is present (a

reflection of fetal distress), it should be taken as hint of impending scar dehiscence.

Remember that the patient may not be in a position to conceive again, and if the baby be born with severe asphyxia, is it easy to raise a special child? A timely LSCS goes a long way in preventing maternal and fetal morbidity.

Tracing the Ureter during LSCS
(Fig. 10.12a–c)

A downward extension of an LSCS incision (Fig. 10.12a); the patient was taken up for emergency LSCS after the cervix was fully dilated for more than an hour. Now, one can wait as long as there are no FHR decelerations since the second

Fig. 10.11a

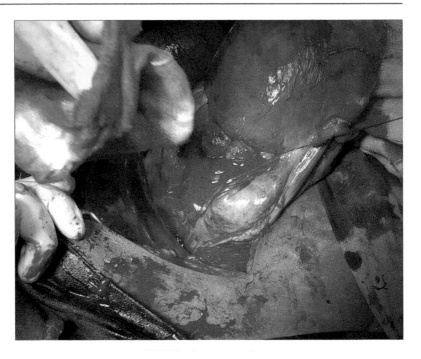

Fig. 10.11b

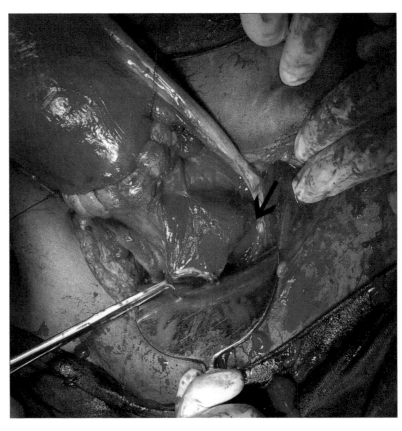

stage of labor in a primipara can take time. But the attending obstetrician must consider

– Is it the vertex? Or is it the caput, which is being felt down below? Are the caput and moulding increasing?
– Could there be loops of cord around the neck? Or a true knot? Or a constriction ring?
– Is the pelvis favorable for baby size?

It can be difficult to deliver the baby when LSCS is done late in the second stage of labor on account of a deeply engaged head. There could be tears in the myometrium, and it may also be necessary to extend the incision upward to convert the transverse lower segment incision into an inverted T- or a J-shaped incision. It may also be difficult to secure hemostasis in such situations.

One can see that the downward extension has been well sutured. The transverse uterine incision and the downward extension have been sutured separately, and then the suture ends have been tied together. When there are extensions, under no circumstances should the entire uterine opening be sutured in a straight line.

There is a stay suture which indicates the lower most point of the extension. But how can one be sure that the ureter has not been injured? There could be blood-stained urine as a result of prolonged second stage and not necessarily due to ureteric or bladder injury.

The obstetrician has exposed the uterine artery with the help of a right-angled forceps. The left hand is on the broad ligament. The sigmoid is located right behind it. So this signifies two things. First, if one takes a deep stitch blindly, a posterior structure like the sigmoid can get included into the stitch and will lead to disastrous consequences. There are cautery burn marks on the broad ligament. One must place one's hand behind the broad ligament to protect the posterior structure before the bleeding points are cauterized, lest the sigmoid also suffers a cautery burn. Since most LSCS are done under spinal anesthesia, the patient could be pushing if the LSCS is being done in the second stage of labor. Bowel

Fig. 10.11c

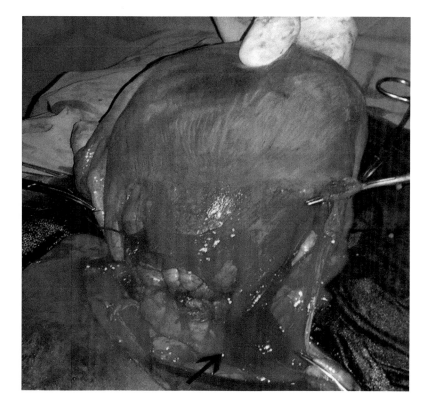

loops may be coming in the way of suturing, and the obstetrician has to be careful not to injure it.

Second, should there be a rent in the broad ligament, it should be closed, lest a loop of bowel projects through it in the postoperative period and results in an internal hernia.

In the above example, the obstetrician must confirm if the ureter is fine before closing. The hemostasis achieved is satisfactory.

The obstetrician is giving gentle traction to the stay suture on the lowest point of the downward extension, as shown by the arrow pointing up (Fig. 10.12b). The horizontal arrow is showing the ureter. As one can see, it is away from the sutures and is intact. The uterine artery has been ligated and cut. The ureter is the "water under the bridge." Though the ureter is away from the sutures, it is not very far. Had the extension been longer, it would have gone beyond the course of the ureter and suturing the extension would have injured it.

So how to differentiate the uterine artery which can be very big during pregnancy, from the ureter? Both can be of the same caliber. Before one ligates or cuts anything, one must confirm the ureter by feeling it—it is like a cord that slips between fingers—and also by looking for peristalsis. The other structure in question has to be

a vessel. In case the structure has been traumatized and one can see blood pouring out, it has to be a blood vessel; just hold the edges and ligate both ends. (Hope the vessel in question is not the external iliac artery! Place a mop and call a vascular surgeon quickly. When dealing with traumatic PPH encountered during LSCS, bleeding vessels are around the lower segment—uterine artery and its branches.)

Similarly, if blood-stained watery fluid is seen coming out of the lumen, then the structure is either the ureter or the bladder. In case of a bladder rent, one can see the tip of the Foley catheter through the rent. But if one finds watery blood collecting in the pelvis, and the tip of Foley catheter is not seen, one can do retrograde filling of the bladder with methylene blue-stained saline. If there is an outpouring of bluish saline in the pelvis, then bladder is certainly injured. Maybe the bladder rent is very small and not easily noticeable.

But if the bladder fills up and one still finds watery bleeding (not methylene blue stained) in the pelvis, then one must trace the ureters on both sides [4, 5]. In all probability, the ureter has been injured. To do this, one has to divide the round ligament quickly but gently locate the ureter. It will be seen running medially along the fold of

Fig. 10.12a

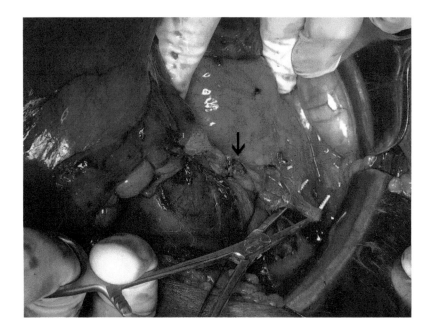

broad ligament. Visible peristalsis or feeling a cord that slips between fingers is confirmatory. The dome of the bladder can be sutured by the obstetrician, but any rent in the posterior wall of bladder or ureteric injury should be repaired by a urologist.

Unless the patient is a case who has been referred very late and has been taken up for LSCS promptly, the obstetrician must review his/her clinical judgment, should ureteric and bladder injuries occur.

A close-up view (Fig. 10.12c) of the previous case showing how close the lower most point of the downward extension is to the ureter. The arrow pointing to the right is pointing the ureter, which fortunately has not been injured or included in the stitches. The arrow pointing to the left is indicating the sigmoid which is behind the fold of the broad ligament.

B-Lynch Suture-Problems (Fig. 10.13)

Figure 10.13 is an image from a patient who had undergone LSCS a few days back and was referred in a state of sepsis. The LSCS wound was full of foul smelling discharge. There was complete wound dehiscence—burst abdomen.

Burst abdomen can happen even in transverse incisions [6, 7]. In the OT, the uterus was full of necrotic slough. One can see there is slough over the uterine incision. The arrow pointing up is showing a fairly big opening below the uterine incision. There was a lot of necrotic material and slough which was removed by repeated saline irrigation. In such situations, it is better not to do any destructive surgery—just drain all pus and debris, irrigate with copious amount of saline, and close with drain.

One can also see that a vertical incision has been taken. This was done since there was a lot of pus in the peritoneal cavity which could not be drained through the same LSCS incision. The patient ended up having an inverted T incision.

The arrow pointing down is showing marks of B-Lynch suture. The referring notes mentioned that there was PPH for which B-Lynch sutures were applied.

Though B-Lynch suture can be applied quickly, one has to consider whether the patient is stable or fast deteriorating? Should one proceed to do uterine artery ligation only if B-Lynch sutures fails to control hemorrhage? And should one proceed to do bilateral internal iliac artery ligation only if bilateral uterine artery ligation fails to con-

Fig. 10.12b

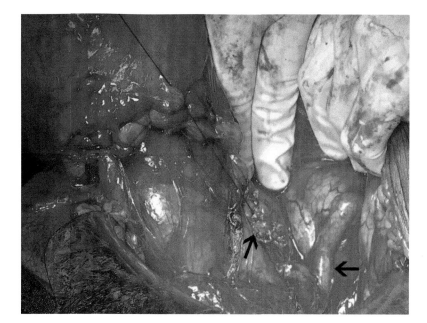

Fig. 10.12c

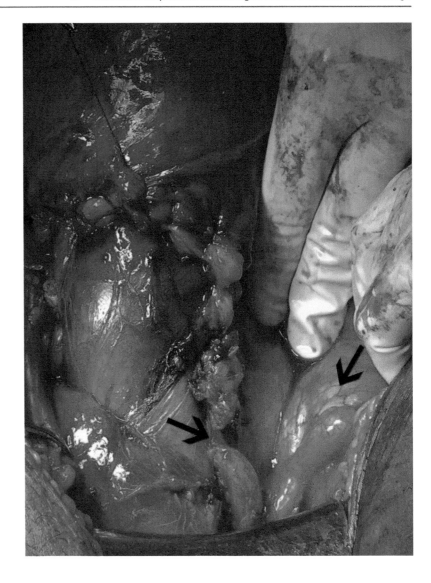

Fig. 10.13

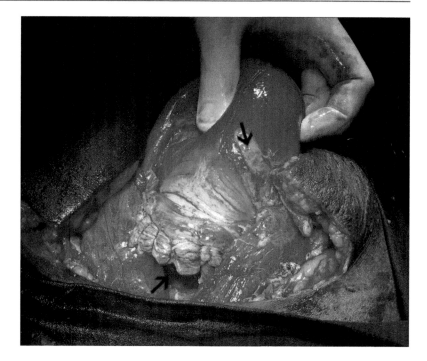

trol hemorrhage? And should one finally do an obstetric hysterectomy only if bilateral internal iliac artery ligation fails to control hemorrhage? Does the condition of the patient permit stepwise devascularization, or should one directly proceed to do caesarean hysterectomy? The obstetrician should decide fast.

References

1. Khadilkar AV, Kajale NA. Bone health status in Indian women. Indian J Med Res. 2013;137(1):7–9.
2. Revicky V, Mukhopadhyay S, Morris EP, Nieto JJ. Can we predict shoulder dystocia? Arch Gynecol Obstet. 2012;285(2):291–5.
3. Broady AJ, Bartholomew ML. Structural umbilical cord and placental abnormalities. Donald School J Ultrasound Obstet Gynecol. 2016;10(1):23–6.
4. Engelsgjerd JS, LaGrange CA. Ureteral injury. Treasure Island: StatPearls Publishing; 2018.
5. Burks FN, Santucci RA. Management of iatrogenic ureteral injury. Ther Adv Urol. 2014;6(3):115–24.
6. Esmat ME. A new technique in closure of burst abdomen TI, TIE and TIES incisions. World J Surg. 2006;30:1063–73.
7. Fleischer GM, Rennert A, Rühmer M. Infected abdominal wall and burst abdomen. Chirurg. 2000;71:754–62.

Internal Iliac Artery Ligation: *Two Different Approaches*

11

Internal iliac artery ligation is a life-saving and, during postpartum hemorrhage, a uterus-saving procedure since it has no effect on future fertility or menstrual function [1]. This is probably because that internal iliac artery ligation helps control pelvic hemorrhage by greatly reducing the pulse pressure and not stopping blood flow entirely. Ligating the anterior division of the artery on both sides should theoretically stop blood flow through the superior and inferior vesical arteries since both arise from the anterior division. But there have been no reports of bladder necrosis or dysfunction either. This is because of the rich anastomosis in the pelvis [1–4]. Embolization of pelvic and uterine vessels by angiographic techniques can also be done to control pelvic hemorrhage. However, this depends on the availability of an intervention radiologist. And the angiographic uterine artery embolization in the setting of PPH (as opposed to embolization for leiomyoma) is associated with loss of circulation to lower extremities, labial and buttock necrosis, and vesicovaginal fistula in 3–5% of cases.

The technique of internal iliac artery ligation entirely depends on the ability of the obstetrician-gynecologist to quickly and correctly locate the bifurcation of the common iliac artery.

There are two ways to do it. The first approach involves dividing the round ligaments and opening the two folds of the broad ligament. The loose areolar tissues are quickly separated, and the iliac vessels are exposed right up to the bifurcation of the common iliac artery. All the structures should now be clearly visible—the common iliac artery with the ureter crossing it over its bifurcation, the external iliac artery which follows a long straight downward course and continues as the femoral artery in the lower limb. There is a blue vessel, much larger in caliber just under the external iliac artery which is the external iliac vein. And there will be a short vessel, the medial branch of the common iliac artery which runs a very short course of about 2 cm and immediately divides into the anterior and posterior divisions [2]. The gynecologist has to quickly gain access to this space without damaging any structure. In case of an LSCS, there will be dilated engorged ovarian vessels that might get damaged and lead to profuse bleeding in an already hemorrhaging patient.

Once the vessels are exposed, one must correctly identify the internal iliac artery. The vessels are seen pulsating, but ureter shows peristalsis. One must not ligate the external iliac artery or the ureter in the heat of the moment.

To ligate the internal iliac artery, a right-angled forceps is gently passed under it about 2 cm from the bifurcation of the common iliac artery. The internal iliac artery can be held or stabilized with a Babcock or a blunt forceps. The artery is lifted gently, without traumatizing the internal iliac vein. If veins are traumatized, dark red blood will be seen pouring out and this will

© Springer Nature Singapore Pte Ltd. 2020
A. R. Podder, J. G Seshadri, *Atlas of Difficult Gynecological Surgery*,
https://doi.org/10.1007/978-981-13-8173-7_11

only worsen the situation. A point where one can pass the right-angled forceps under the internal iliac artery is chosen. The assistant can feed a stout linen or silk into the right-angled forceps. The suture is tied preferably with sliding hand knots; not only is the situation an emergency, there will be many engorged vessels which can get traumatized if one tries to tie the knot with the needle holder. But if using a needle holder or an artery forceps to ligate, avoid taking the instrument close to the engorged vessels, lest they get traumatized. Because one is under a lot of stress, one must not apply so much energy to tie the knots that the ligature snaps. The iliac veins can get traumatized and will worsen the situation, if one repeatedly tries to pass the right-angled forceps under the internal iliac artery.

The procedure must be repeated on the other side. The area should be mopped and gentle pressure applied to check if bleeding is still persisting. One must doubly check if the wrong structure has been ligated. If external iliac artery is ligated, there will be no lower limb pulses—femoral, popliteal, posterior tibial, and dorsalis pedis will not be felt or will be very feeble if the ligature is not tight. The best medico-legal safety measure is to ask for another pulse oximeter and check for lower limb pulses and oxygen saturation. If both the pulse rate and the oxygen saturation in the lower limb are identical to that of upper limb, then one can conclude that the external iliac artery has not been ligated. Urine must be checked for hematuria, urine can be blood tinged due to handling and not necessarily due to ureteric injury.

This method, in author's experience, is suitable for gynecological surgeries, especially during radical surgeries or when there is profuse hemorrhage in case of surgeries for large leiomyomas—myomectomy or hysterectomy. But in case of LSCS, one can approach the internal iliac artery through another route which gives faster access to the iliac vessels. The uterus is big even after delivery of the baby, about 24 weeks size, and the surrounding tissues are edematous and congested. Dividing the round ligaments and then trying to gain access to the axilla of the pelvis might itself lead to further

bleeding if the engorged vessels are damaged. Also, bowels may be dilated, and the patient may be pushing/bearing down if she has been taken up in advanced labor. The visualization through a Pfannenstiel incision may not be adequate. One must ask for general anesthesia, and convert the Pfannenstiel incision to Maylard incision by extending the skin incision and dividing the rectus muscle. Ask for another assistant, exteriorize the uterus, and expose the pouch of Douglas. Hold the fold of peritoneum on the pouch of Douglas and make sure there is no structure underneath by feeling with thumb and index finger. Cauterize it and open the retroperitoneal space. Remember that the ureter is present along the fold of the broad ligament; it passes under the uterine artery to enter the tunnel of Wertheim. Feel the ureter with thumb and index finger and cut the peritoneum little by little.

By opening the pouch of Douglas, one can get quick access to the axilla of the pelvis—the bifurcation of the common iliac artery with the ureter crossing it. Make sure to correctly identify the structure. Pass a stout thread under the internal iliac artery with the help of a right-angled forceps, and tie it on both sides quickly and check if any wrong structure has been ligated in excitement and tension.

If the internal iliac artery ligation is done, it is advisable to close the abdomen with a drain in pouch of Douglas and give DVT prophylaxis from the second day of surgery. This should be done irrespective of whether internal iliac artery ligation was done in a gynecological surgery or following delivery. Drain is like a window and can tell what is happening inside the peritoneal cavity—*Is the patient still bleeding?* Pelvic surgery is a known risk factor for DVT and pregnancy is a known hypercoagulable state [5].

In case of profuse hemorrhage during laparoscopic surgeries, the ability to perform internal iliac artery ligation depends on many factors like obesity, difficulty level of the case, etc. When in doubt or when not having able assistants, one must convert the case into a laparotomy. The decision of taking a vertical or transverse incision depends on the difficulty level of the case. A transverse Maylard incision should work fine for internal iliac artery ligation alone.

But to perform the procedure laparoscopically, one must expose the bifurcation of common iliac artery by dividing the round ligament, and split open the two folds of broad ligament with a hook. Hold a small fold of the peritoneum with a grasper and lift it and cauterize it to enter the retroperitoneal space. Once the structures are exposed and identified, clips can be directly applied on the internal iliac artery using a clip applicator. The procedure is repeated on the other side, and one must check once again whether clips have been applied on the wrong structure.

Let us now study the photographs taken during live surgery, where sudden profuse bleeding was encountered and internal iliac artery ligation had to be done.

How to Locate the Internal Iliac Artery? (Fig. 11.1)

The round ligament has been cut; the two folds of broad ligament have been divided (Fig. 11.1). The loose areolar tissue has been cleared to expose the iliac vessels and the ureter. The ureter shows peristalsis when stimulated with a blunt forceps. The external iliac artery runs a straight downward course to become the formoral artery in the lower limb, and it is the longer of the two branches of common iliac artery. The external iliac vein will be located just below the external iliac artery. The internal iliac artery on the other hand is the short medial branch of the common iliac artery.

Internal Iliac Artery Ligation Accomplished (Fig. 11.2)

Internal iliac artery ligation has been accomplished (Fig. 11.2). Arrow 1 shows the ureter. If it is traced upwards, it can be seen crossing the bifurcation of the common iliac artery.

Arrow 2 shows the internal iliac artery at the point where it has been ligated. With the help of a right-angled forceps, stout silk was passed under the internal iliac artery, and it has been ligated.

Arrow 3 is pointing at the bifurcation of the common iliac artery. If the external iliac artery is ligated in the heat of the moment, one can imagine the disastrous consequences that will follow.

Fig. 11.1

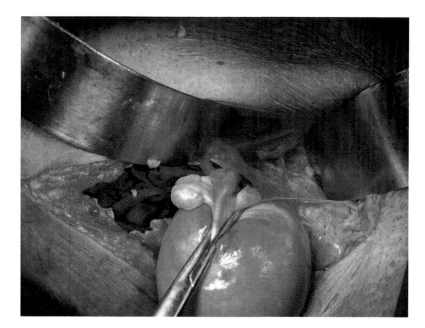

Fig. 11.2

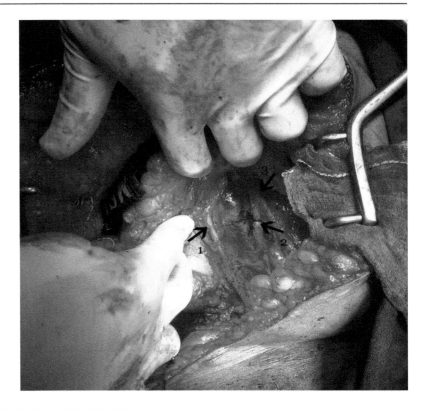

Approaching the Internal Iliac Artery through the Pouch of Douglas (Fig. 11.3a–d)

Proceeding to do the internal iliac artery ligation for PPH—approaching the internal iliac artery through the pouch of Douglas (Fig. 11.3a).

The baby has been delivered by LSCS. The pouch of Douglas is being opened to gain access to the iliac vessels. One can imagine the difficulty if one approaches the internal iliac artery by dividing the round ligament in a postpartum uterus. There will be congested and engorged vessels which can get easily traumatized and cause further bleeding.

A fold of the peritoneum has been held with a forceps. It will be opened to gain access to the retroperitoneal space.

Gently developing the posterior space after opening the pouch of Douglas (Fig. 11.3b).

Rough handling could traumatize the thin-walled veins, leading to obscuring of the operating field, worsening an already precarious situation.

The posterior space has been opened, and now the iliac vessels are seen (Fig. 11.3c). One has to correctly locate the internal iliac and the external iliac artery and the ureter. The consequences of ligating the ureter or the external iliac cannot be underestimated. While incising the peritoneum, one must feel the peritoneum with thumb and index finger; make sure that the ureter is not present underneath before incising it.

The ureter has been located prior to ligating the internal iliac artery by the pouch of Douglas approach (Fig. 11.3d). It is seen coursing along the fold of broad ligament. Feel it with thumb and index finger; it will feel like a cord that slips between the fingers. Or gently stimulate it with a blunt forceps; presence of peristalsis confirms that the structure is the ureter.

Now that the ureter has been excluded and the internal iliac artery correctly identified, pass a stout silk or linen under it with the help of a right-angled forceps and tie it.

Fig. 11.3a

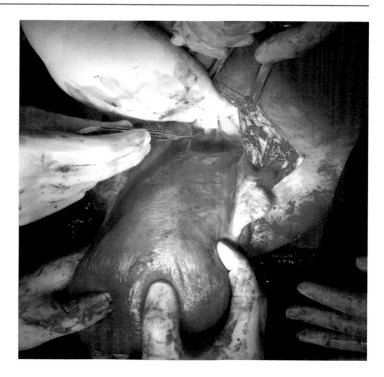

Fig. 11.3b

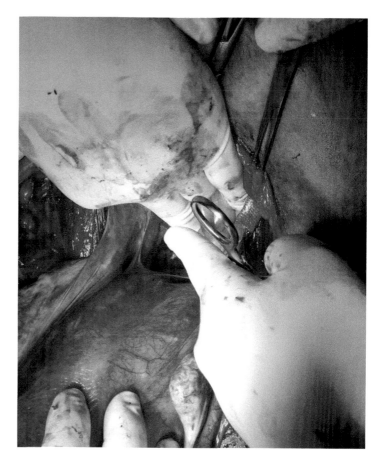

Fig. 11.3c

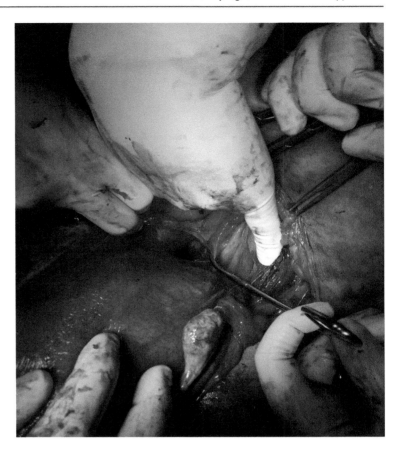

Fig. 11.3d

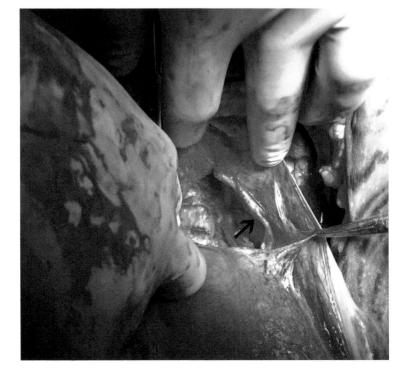

References

1. Mukhopadhyay P, Naskar T, Hazra S, Bhattacharya D. Emergency internal iliac artery ligation - still a life saving procedure. J Obstet Gynaecol India. 2005;55(2):144–5.
2. Sakthivelavan S, Sendiladdiban DS, Jebakkani CF. Multiple variations of internal iliac artery-case report. J Anat Soc India. 2014;63:89–91.
3. Bellad MB. Internal iliac artery ligation (IIAL): a uterus/life saving procedure. J SAFOG. 2009;1(2):32–3.
4. Singh A, Kishore R, Saxena SS. Ligating internal iliac artery: success beyond hesitation. J Obstet Gynaecol India. 2016;66(Suppl 1):235–41.
5. Mclendon K, Attia M. Deep venous thrombosis (DVT), risk factors. StatPearls [internet]. Last update: 1 March 2019.

Abdominal Closure and Burst Abdomen: *Poor Wound Healing Can Ruin Everything*

12

Most of the gynecological surgeries are either done through a transverse incision or laparoscopically. The closure of transverse incisions and laparoscopic port sites is easy. Transverse incision by nature tends to heal [1]. This is because the blood supply to the wound margins is better when the incision is taken transversely. Also, when a person coughs, sneezes, or vomits, the increased intra-abdominal pressure tends to separate the sutures maximally, around the umbilicus and in the midline. Therefore, small incisions (laparoscopic port sites) and lower abdominal transverse incisions are less likely to gape. However, one must keep in mind that burst abdomen is known to occur even in transverse incisions [2–4]. Incisional hernia is known to occur even in laparoscopic port site incisions. The author has had one experience where the infraumbilical laparoscopic wound had got infected, and on the tenth postoperative day, the rectus sutures had given away. One could see the omentum and the small intestines through the infraumbilical wound. Wound infection around the umbilicus particularly tends to be painful and disfiguring in nature.

However, the challenge of abdominal closure is mainly concerning vertical incision since the complications of wound gape, burst abdomen, and hernia are more commonly associated with it. Obesity, diabetes mellitus, and history of previous chemotherapy and previous radiation to abdomen increase the chances of wound gape.

Other systemic factors like anemia, nutritional deficiencies, chronic renal failure, liver failure, prolonged corticosteroid use, all adversely affect wound healing [5–7].

In case of a transverse incision, the author prefers to close the rectus sheath preferably with a nonabsorbable suture followed by subcuticular closure of the skin with an absorbable suture. The peritoneum is not sutured, and the rectus muscle is not sutured even when it has been cut as in case of a Maylard incision. In case of re-suturing of a wound gape, or in cases of primary closure of the wound in obese patients, skin is closed with vertical mattress sutures with a drain in situ. Drain in subcutaneous space is also preferred in all patients with bleeding disorders to prevent collection of blood and serous fluid in the subcutaneous space [8]. Staples can also be used for skin closure, but unlike subcuticular closure, the patient needs to come back after discharge for staple removal, or the patient has to stay in the hospital till the staples are removed.

For laparoscopic surgeries, closure of the rectus sheath in the camera port site is a must, since this is 10 mm and around the umbilicus - the point where there is maximum separating force during coughing, sneezing, straining, vomiting, or any act which increases intra-abdominal pressure.

Hopefully, the earlier chapters of this book have convinced the readers about the fact that a vertical incision sometimes extending above the

© Springer Nature Singapore Pte Ltd. 2020
A. R. Podder, J. G Seshadri, *Atlas of Difficult Gynecological Surgery*,
https://doi.org/10.1007/978-981-13-8173-7_12

umbilicus is still required for many situations in modern-day gynecological practice. This is because laparoscopy has a long learning curve and robotic surgeries are not going to be easily accessible to all sections of society anytime soon.

The author prefers to close the vertical incision in layers. The peritoneum is closed with absorbable suture material, followed by the rectus sheath which is closed using a nonabsorbable material. The skin is closed using staplers, and a drain is placed in the subcutaneous space if the subcutaneous fat is thick. The logic behind this method is that in case of mass closure, a single suture is responsible for the integrity of the closure. Should it give way at any one point (let us say due to tissue necrosis or infection), it will result in burst abdomen [9]. But if the abdomen is closed in layers and if the rectus sheath gives way at any point, the closed peritoneum will technically still hold the abdominal wall. It will prevent evisceration and burst abdomen. Peritoneum is a tissue which heals very fast, but it is unlikely to close by itself within a week if bowels are constantly coming in contact with the sutures above or if there is raised intra-abdominal pressure. However, if the risk factors for burst abdomen (cough, abdominal distention due to paralytic ileus, full bladder, straining due to constipation and vomiting, anything that causes increased abdominal pressure) are not controlled in the postoperative period, there is a high risk of burst abdomen irrespective of the type of abdominal closure.

A drain is always placed in the abdomen to keep the intra-abdominal collection low. Following lymphadenectomy, extensive dissection, or in cases of pelvic abscess, there can be significant collection in the peritoneal cavity. The drain serves as a window; should there be a bowel perforation that has been missed, presence of feculent and/or bile-stained drain fluid in the drain output will help in its prompt detection. A drain, by virtue of keeping the collection low, prevents the air-filled intestines from floating and coming in contact with the abdominal sutures above.

The subcutaneous drain keeps the collection in the subcutaneous space low and removes the

nidus for infection [8]. Sudden increase in the output of the subcutaneous drain is probably a harbinger of burst abdomen, especially if the drain fluid of pelvic and subcutaneous drains is identical.

In both vertical and transverse incisions, subcutaneous fat is not closed even in very obese patients. Catgut is a suture material that should never be used in any part of abdominal closure. Because of its low cost, it is continued to be used for episiotomy closure in our country, though technically it is not a good choice.

Whenever the author has encountered burst abdomen, the abdomen was immediately closed after thoroughly irrigating the peritoneal cavity with copious amounts of saline and placing a drain in the pouch of Douglas.

The general condition of the patient usually does not permit a layered closure, and it is usually not possible to close the peritoneum because edges are frayed, and they will cut through. In addition, bowels are dilated, and unless general anesthesia is given (the anesthetists might be reluctant since the general condition will be poor in most cases. Most patients will be obese and diabetic and would have undergone a long surgery about a week earlier.), it may not be possible to relax the abdomen. The abdomen is closed using nonabsorbable sutures in an interrupted manner. The sutures are placed one at a time from above and below (taking sutures on the upper end and the lower end of the incision, and gradually coming to the midpoint from both ends). After 2–3 sutures are placed, the assistant places his palm below to depress the bowels while the surgeon lifts the two ends of the suture and ties it. This ensures that a loop of bowel is not entrapped in one of the sutures. After closing the incision from above and below, the last stitch is placed midway, taking care that bites have not been taken through any visceral structure. The reason for taking time-consuming interrupted sutures over continuous sutures to close burst abdomen is that the wound margins are frayed and have poor blood supply; they may cut through unless a good chunk of tissue is taken. So even if one of the interrupted sutures gives way, the rest of the sutures should still be intact provided there is no increase in abdominal pressure postoperatively. It is very important to control cough (think respiratory infection), and vomiting (think electrolyte imbalance—hyponatremia) in the postoperative period [10]. The role of postoperative chest physiotherapy should not be seen as a cursory routine. It helps in expelling chest secretions.

In the postoperative period, anemia, diabetes, hypoproteinemia, and electrolyte imbalance should be aggressively corrected. There should be no hurry to start oral sips, in all cases where there was extensive bowel handling, para-aortic dissection (which can cause delayed return of bowel activity due to handling of hypogastric plexus), and also following closure of burst abdomen. The author prefers to start oral sips only after the patient passes flatus and ensuring that there is no hypokalemia and hyponatremia. Hypokalemia is associated with paralytic ileus which causes distention which is associated with burst abdomen [11]. Hyponatremia is associated with vomiting, which if uncorrected can further worsen hyponatremia.

In addition to taking measures to prevent raised intra-abdominal pressure in the postoperative period, a corset dressing can be applied in obese patients who have a pendulous abdomen that sways from side to side. This helps in stabilizing the panniculus and reduces the stress on the sutures due to the movement of the panniculus. The skin sutures will be subject to separating forces if the thick pad of fat keeps moving; continuous movement will prevent collagen fibers from bridging the wound.

A corset dressing is applied in the following manner. The wound dressing is done in the usual way, and this is followed by applying 2–3 patches of elastic bandage on either flank. Fenestrations are made inside the patches. Roller gauze is applied from fenestration of one side to the other and tied in the middle, taking care that there is enough slack. The patient will find it very difficult to breathe if there is too much of tension.

As compared to an abdominal binder, corset can be applied according to the position of the drains. The gauze can be loosened and retied accordingly. The problem with the use of a binder

is that it gets dirty and acts like a fomite. But a corset dressing is discarded and a new dressing applied daily or whenever required. Also, a binder becomes loose in most patients since they also suffer from a poor appetite and lose weight in the postoperative period.

The main disadvantage of the corset is that the some patients develop skin excoriation due to prolonged use of elastic bandage. This however is a temporary problem and resolves quickly.

How to Apply a Corset Dressing
(Fig. 12.1a–f)

The wound has been dressed with elastic bandage in the usual way (Fig. 12.1a). There is a drain placed in the subcutaneous space and also in the peritoneal cavity. This patient has undergone laparotomy for ovarian torsion five days before. After surgery, the wound was dressed followed by the application of corset. Now the dressing has been changed. The author prefers doing a check dressing usually 96 h after laparotomy. Now, a new corset will be applied.

Elastic patches have been applied on the flank, and fenestrations have been made in them (Fig. 12.1b).

A roller gauze has been threaded through the fenestrations from one side to the other (Fig. 12.1c). A pad has been placed in the center to cushion the sutures. The position of the drain has been kept in mind while applying the elastic patches on the flanks and threading the roller gauze. After tying the roller gauze, there should be enough slack so that the patient can breathe comfortably, and at the same time, the gauze must be tied tight enough to provide support and stabilize the panniculus.

A corset dressing has been applied (Fig. 12.1d). This can be changed as and when required till the suture/staple removal is complete

A corset dressing seen from the side (Fig. 12.1e).

One can appreciate the obesity and the pendulous nature of the abdomen. The sutures would be subjected to continuous separating forces if the side-to-side movement of the anterior abdominal fat is not stopped. In other words, the

Fig. 12.1a

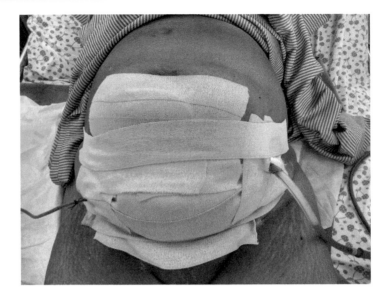

Fig. 12.1b

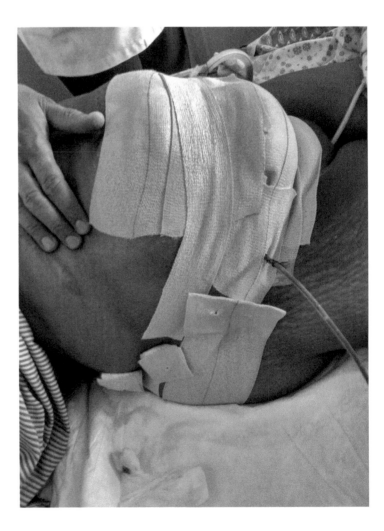

Fig. 12.1c

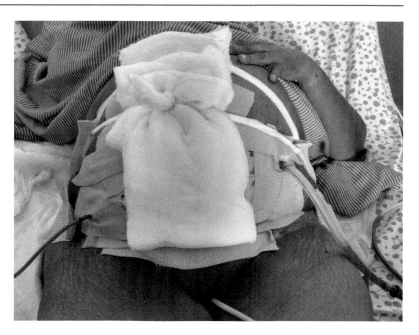

Fig. 12.1d

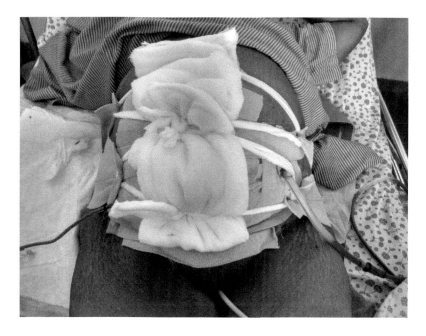

Fig. 12.1e

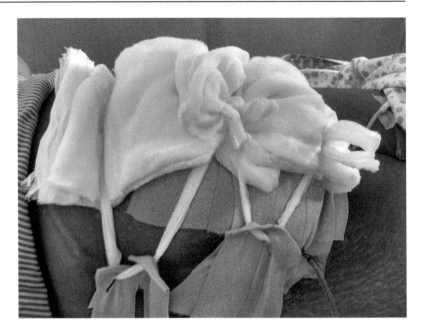

Fig. 12.1f

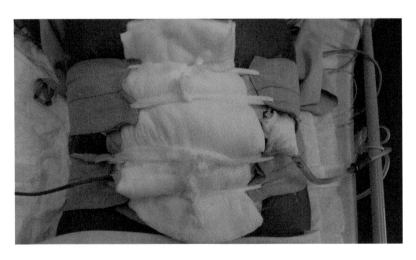

panniculus has to be stabilized. The drain tubes are free, not kinked. The collected fluid can freely flow out.

The stabilizing effect of a corset can be appreciated (Fig. 12.1f).

The patient appears to have lost some weight. This image is on day 10 of laparotomy. Check dressing has been done on day 5, and the dressing is being changed every alternate day. Perspiration and moisture tend to collect especially during the hot months. If one observes carefully, it can be seen that the wound has been dressed with micropore dressing. The corset has been applied with elastic bandage.

A Healthy Wound (Fig. 12.2)

The dressing and the corset have just been removed. It is day 14 of laparotomy (Fig. 12.2). The wound margins are healthy with no induration. Staples can now be removed.

Fig. 12.2

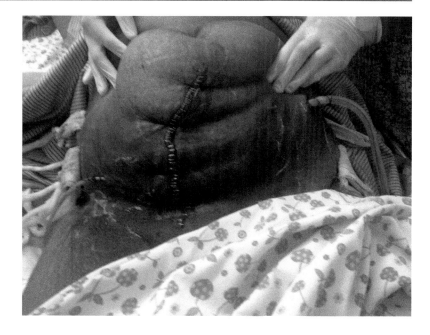

References

1. Grantcharov TP, Rosenberg J. Vertical compared with transverse incisions in abdominal surgery. Eur J Surg. 2001;167(4):260–7.
2. Esmat ME. A new technique in closure of burst abdomen TI, TIE and TIES incisions. World J Surg. 2006;30:1063–73.
3. Fleischer GM, Rennert A, Ruᵎhmer M. Infected abdominal wall and burst abdomen. Chirurg. 2000;71:754–62.
4. Walming S, et al. Retrospective review of risk factors for surgical wound dehiscence and incisional hernia. BMC Surg. 2017;17:19.
5. Payne WG, et al. Wound healing in patients with cancer. Eplasty. 2008;8:e9.
6. Gieringer M, Gosepath J, Naim R. Radiotherapy and wound healing: principles, management and prospects. Oncol Rep. 2011;26:299–307.
7. Guo S, DiPietro LA. Factors affecting wound healing. J Dent Res. 2010;89(3):219–29.
8. Manzoor B, Heywood N, Sharma A. Review of subcutaneous wound drainage in reducing surgical site infections after laparotomy. Surg Res Pract. 2015;2015:715803.
9. Deshmukh SN, Maske AN. Mass closure versus layered closure of midline laparotomy incisions: a prospective comparative study. Int Surg J. 2018;5(2):584–7.
10. Sahay M, Sahay R. Hyponatremia: a practical approach. Indian J Endocrinol Metab. 2014;18(6):760–71.
11. Berge NG, Ridolfi TJ, Ludwig KA. Delayed gastrointestinal recovery after abdominal operation—role of alvimopan. Clin Exp Gastroenterol. 2015;8:231–5.